Stephen Griffiths was plagued with ill health caused by an overload of allergies and toxins in his system. His worsening condition forced him to retire from his position as a director of one of Australia's largest real estate companies. Unaided by doctors in this country Stephen had to reconcile himself to his chronic ill health or seek help overseas. On the invitation of Dr Julian N. Kenyon he went to England where finally his allergies were diagnosed and treated.

Gradually, through the help of Dr Kenyon and his own sound management of food and chemical allergy problems, Stephen has been restored to good health. Once again he is actively involved in his profession as a real estate agent and property developer in Western Australia.

During his recuperation his interest in the damaging effect of allergies on the body intensified. This book is the result of the extensive research he has made into all aspects of allergies and his assessment of the current medical theories about their treatment and causes.

ALLERGY OVERLOAD

STEPHEN GRIFFITHS

A division of HarperCollins*Publishers*

AN ANGUS & ROBERTSON BOOK

First published in Australia by William Collins Pty Ltd in 1987
Reprinted in 1987 (three times), 1988
This corrected edition published by Collins/Angus & Robertson
Publishers Australia in 1990

Collins/Angus & Robertson Publishers Australia
A division of HarperCollinsPublishers (Australia) Pty Limited
Unit 4, Eden Park, 31 Waterloo Road, North Ryde
NSW 2113, Australia

William Collins Publishers Ltd
31 View Road, Glenfield, Auckland 10, New Zealand

Angus & Robertson (UK)
16 Golden Square, London W1R 4BN, United Kingdom

National Library of Australia
Cataloguing-in-Publication data:

Griffiths, Stephen.
    Allergy overload.

    Bibliography.
    Includes index

    ISBN 0 207 17074 6

    I. Allergy. 2. Allergy -- Diagnosis. 3. Drug
    allergy 4. Food allergy. I. Title.

616.97

Typeset by Press Etching (Qld.) Pty Ltd., Brisbane
Printed by The Book Printer, Victoria

 10 9   8   7   6
95 94 93 92 91 90

For Helen, with love

Acknowledgements

I wish to acknowledge the help I have had from several people, before and during the course of writing this book. Dr J.L. Quintner, Rheumatologist, of Perth, Western Australia; for having the magnanimity to suggest the possibility of multiple allergies. Professor C. Stewart Goodwin, Associate Professor in Clinical Microbiology and Head of Department of Microbiology, Royal Perth Hospital; for his diagnosis, his help and his research into multiple allergy illness. Ria Plate, past Secretary of the Myalgic Encephalomyelitis Society in Western Australia; for her untiring efforts to help others. Dr Julian N. Kenyon of Southampton and London, Clinical Ecologist, researcher and practitioner of Environmental Medicine, humanitarian and doctor extraordinaire; his great knowledge, foresight and understanding sets him apart from his peers. Helene Schroeder, English teacher, Christian and friend; for her linguistic assistance in preparing the final draft of this book. Helen Ann O'Grady, teacher, actress, business partner and loving wife; whose love, tenderness and understanding gave me the will and made it possible.

Foreword

It is an honour to be asked to write a foreword to such a complete book on ecological illness. It remains an enigma that such an important new area of medicine, which has more recently become known as environmental medicine, should be attracting so much interest from the general public and so little from the medical profession. This book is a timely reminder to the medical profession that it ought to take a more serious look at the effects of the environment on patients' health. Even more so because this book hasn't been written by a doctor, but by an extremely well-informed layman, who has himself suffered and has subsequently sorted himself out, largely by looking at his environment. I feel sure that this book will help many sufferers, in that it is readable, practical and easy to follow. The ecological approach is completely harmless, but can sort out many intractable problems, which may have been untreatable, or requiring potentially dangerous suppressive drug treatment in order to control the symptoms. I am certain that many people will find this book not only interesting but of real practical use in many chronic illnesses. Most of all I hope it attracts the interest of the medical profession, and for them to be humble enough to acknowledge that they have been prodded to take an interest in the environment by their patients and not by their colleagues.

Dr Julian N. Kenyon, M.D., M.B., CH.B.
Southampton and London,
July 1985

Preface

It is because good medical help for allergies is so very difficult to find that I decided to write this book. My experiences over many years with my own masked food and chemical allergies have shown me that the best physician for this problem is oneself. In my case I was fortunate to be able to travel to Britain and consult one of the best specialists in environmental medicine available — Dr Julian Kenyon of Southampton and Harley Street, London. He was able to diagnose my allergies and point me in the right direction for eventual return to good health. When I returned to Australia, I realized that in order to stay on top of this illness, one needed to understand it, and that meant learning as much about allergies and ecological disease as possible.

In my search for information, I came to realize that a book was needed, in layman's language, which would give the widest possible view of food and chemical allergy illness. Why? Because people need as much information as possible to understand the disease. Recovery is dependent upon effective self-management and without adequate knowledge this is impossible. Therefore, it is important to know more than just the causes, one must determine the reasons for the causes. It is necessary to know how and why the body is affected, and to understand why doctors are not diagnosing this problem. Above all, it is necessary to know what can be done about it, by oneself, because effective self-management can restore a level of good health which you would have never dreamed possible. I feel that the information offered here will enable fellow sufferers to achieve just that. In other words, I have attempted to put together information which I would have dearly loved to come across during the many frustrating years when nobody could tell me what was going wrong with my body.

I have made several criticisms of the medical profession in this book which I am sure I will be taken to task for. They are not meant to include the hardworking and caring doctors who are making an effort to understand the food and chemical allergy problem. Sadly, these are far too few. Generally speaking, the medical profession has settled into a self-complacent rut. Scientific and surgical advancement in specialised fields has over-shadowed the urgent need for clinical reform. As our first line of defence, general practitioners in particular are at fault. They rely too heavily on modern drugs which wreak biochemical havoc in the body and prepetuate illness whilst palliating symptoms. As a result, many people are suffering unfairly, yet there is ample information available to help prevent this.

It is important to remember that a growing number of people, perhaps 20 per cent of the population, are now suffering from continuing distress due to food and chemical allergy symptoms. By the end of the century, as many as 50 per cent may be suffering from these problems to some degree. It is important, therefore, that people begin to appreciate the problem if they want to avoid a lifetime of illness and discomfort. To this end, people must become their own physicians. The more information produced on this subject, in a helpful and readable manner, the better it will be for the population at large. I believe now that many people are looking for information and that many more books will be published in the future, offering a greater understanding of food and chemical allergy illness.

It is advisable to obtain an overview of the food and chemical allergy problems, and so you should read this book completely before applying the appropriate section to your own situation.

S.G.

It appears to me necessary to every physician to be skilled in nature and to strive to know, if he would wish to perform his duties, what man is, in relation to the articles of food and drink and to his other occupations and what are the effects of each of them on everyone. Whoever does not know what effect these things produce upon man cannot know the consequences which result from them. Whoever pays no attention to these things, or paying attention does not comprehend them, how can he understand the diseases which befall man? For by every one of these things man is affected and changed this way and that, and the whole of his life is subject to them — whether in health, convalescence or disease. Nothing else then can be more important and necessary to know than these things.

Hippocrates

CONTENTS

Introduction

PART 1 FOOD AND CHEMICAL ALLERGIES

PART II ALLERGY MANAGEMENT

INTRODUCTION

Several years ago I became very ill. I was in a state of great discomfort and found it impossible to move quickly and think clearly. My body was puffy and my complexion often discoloured. I tended to feel cold when it was hot and hot when it was cold. I ached often and sweated a lot. I found it difficult to concentrate and remember things. I had vision and hearing problems. My digestive system refused to function properly. I could not sleep for more than two hours at a time, yet I was constantly tired. My sinuses plagued me and exertion caused giddiness and exhaustion. I began to confront my own demise.

As a child I had suffered from quite a few health problems which continued into adolescence. Vigorous army service as a young man seemed to build up my health but, after a few years, it started to deteriorate again. Over the years one symptom or another would flare up, while the fatigue and aching became worse. During this time I consulted many doctors but none was able to diagnose the problem. Time and time again I was treated for the symptoms. Antihistamines were prescribed for catarrh, antibiotics for bladder infections, analgesics for aching, cortisone for sinus inflammation, and so on.

During one memorable period, I spent a total of three weeks in various hospitals undergoing every test that a rheumatologist and a neurologist could devise. However, they could not determine what was wrong. At the final consultation, before they washed their hands of me, I was told that a lot of money had been spent on tests and should I ever find out what was wrong would I please let them know. I remember walking out of that consulting room with a feeling of dread and frustration.

In the ensuing weeks I became very depressed. If two top specialists and all those hospital tests could not find out what was wrong with me, then what future did I have? But being a resilient person I decided to fight back. I put myself on a restricted diet and began to run in the morning and to exercise at a health club. I felt a great need to try to rid my body of what seemed to be a constant build up of poisons.

Many times I had complained to doctors and finally to the two venerable specialists, that I felt I was being poisoned. I suspected that somehow my own body was generating poisons which were continually dragging me down and causing me to feel ill. How close I was to the truth! Yet not once did the doctors give credibility to what should have been their patient's most important comment. One doctor, to his credit, did diagnose an airborne allergy problem and I was given a course of injections which, for a while, dampened down my hay fever and sinus problems. The other symptoms, particularly the physical and mental fatigue, the aching, the overheating and the sleeplessness, continued to plague me.

My job as a director of a national real estate company was demanding, but with the additional stress caused by my illness, life became impossible. It reached the point where at the end of the day I could hardly walk the fifty metres to my parked car. I had by this time given up exercise and finally I had to give up my job. For fifteen years I had been ill and I was getting worse.

It was at this time that I came to hear about multiple allergies. Several articles had appeared in the newspaper about people who appeared to have allergies to almost everything. It was being called the 'twentieth century disease'. The articles also suggested that many people in Australia and other Western countries, were beginning to show signs of allergic reactions to their diet and to chemicals and toxins in their environment. Some had become totally incapacitated whilst others appeared to suffer from regular illness and poor health in general.

These articles intrigued me and I began to look for more information on food and chemical allergies. I found that in general, doctors knew very little about this subject and that conventional allergy testing was only really effective for airborne causes such as pollen and house dust. Certainly my experiences had shown that doctors were not tuned in to this problem, as not once had it been suggested to me over the period of fifteen years, that my wide-ranging symptoms were caused by food or chemical allergies.

During this period I also consulted several naturopaths who, while being well-meaning, were not able to prescribe any course of treatment that helped. In fact, in one case the treatment, which consisted of a herbal tonic, made me feel significantly worse. About this time, I was referred to Professor Stewart Goodwin at the Royal Perth Hospital and under his guidance I proceeded to follow a dietary approach. Unfortunately, shortly after, he had to go overseas for six months. There was no time to evaluate the diet and during the next few months my condition became worse. In desperation I contacted several doctors in other parts of Australia and in New Zealand, whom I felt might have had some answers. In each case their response was non-committal and I concluded that they did not have the answers.

My wife, Helen, suggested that I look to treatment overseas. We heard about a clinic in the United States and rang it without delay. We were told that treatment was possible but nothing was guaranteed, and a minimum stay of six weeks would be necessary, at a cost of around $20,000. We started to consider it seriously.

Suddenly some information came our way which changed everything. We heard through the Myalgic Encephalomyelitis (M.E.) Society that there was a highly-qualified doctor in England, specialising in a new branch of medicine, known as 'clinical ecology' which is to do with the effects of diet and the environment on people. His name was Dr Julian Kenyon and he practised in Southampton, as well as having rooms in Harley Street, London. We rang Dr Kenyon, described my problems to him and asked whether he thought he could help. His reply was immediate and positive. He had no doubt that he could help me and we were able to make an appointment for him to see me in Southampton in the following week. Sick though I was, I remember the most incredible uplifting of the spirit after that telephone conversation. His cheerful confidence inspired me. For the first time in years I felt hope for the future.

The following week, I arrived in Southampton and met Julian Kenyon. I found his confidence, energy and incredible alertness of mind a wonderful example of a person who practised what he preached. For four weeks I remained as an outpatient at this clinic. During that time he conducted many tests on me using sophisticated electronic acupuncture equipment, specifically designed for diagnostic purposes.

I was found to be allergic to grains, milk, cheese, chocolate, white sugar, tartrazine (artificial colouring), yeast, fish, shellfish, pork (including ham and bacon), mushrooms, coffee, nuts, cocoa, monosodium glutamate (found in most tinned foods), and tap water (chlorine and fluoride). The milk and grain allergies meant that all products containing these foods were out. The yeast allergy also meant that as well as bread, I would have to stop eating all other yeast-containing foods. Apart from the foods, further testing showed that I was allergic to the lining in tin cans, formalin, petrol, diesel, butane gas and cigarette smoke. Various pollens also showed up as being allergenic.

Perhaps I should have been horrified at the number of allergies diagnosed by Dr Kenyon, but instead I experienced a feeling of the most profound relief, bordering on elation. After all those years of illness, I finally had a positive diagnosis! I was not a hypochondriac, or a psychotic. I was, however, one of a growing number of people who, in this latter part of the twentieth century, has developed wide-ranging sensitivities to foods and chemicals. I was still very sick, my symptoms were worse than they had ever been. The flight from Australia to London had been an ordeal of aching and sleeplessness. On the train trip from Gatwick Airport to Southampton I wondered how it was possible to feel so bad without passing out. Looking back, I suppose there were two reasons. Firstly, my toxin overloaded body would not let me relax enough and secondly, I was determined to get to Southampton as I felt it was my one last chance.

During my stay in Southampton, Dr Kenyon prescribed various homeopathic medicines, which I took before and after meals, designed to help cleanse the body of accumulated toxins. I also had to drink large quantities of distilled water. The effects on the bladder were catastrophic! My forays around Southampton became dependent on nearness to public toilets and other establishments, where they were available. With respect to that aspect of Southampton's geography, I became something of an expert!

The effect of these medicines became noticeable after about a week as I started to lose the terrible toxic heaviness that I had experienced for so long. However, recovery was a slow process. My body had been badly hammered by the build up of toxins over a long period. When one is allergic to a substance, the body becomes poisoned by it and as my diet had consisted of most of the things to which I was allergic, I had been poisoning myself, unknowingly, over a long period of time. These accumulated poisons (or toxins) had caused severe dysfunction in my pancreas, liver and intestine and the result was chaos and chronic ill health.

While the cleansing process was designed to help the overloaded system, the main approach was simply to avoid eating, or coming in contact with, the offending allergenic substances. Accordingly, I began to adjust to a restricted diet that was very different from what I had been used to. Unfortunately it was not just a matter of giving up foods but also of experiencing the withdrawal symptoms that accompany the cessation of eating allergenic foods. The body craves the allergens as an alcoholic craves alcohol, and so the first two weeks were very difficult. However, the last week in Southampton was an exhilarating time. I was still having a lot of ups and downs but the general improvement was so noticeable that nagging symptoms and bad days did not dampen my spirits. I found I had the energy to go for long walks and I knew I had finally turned the corner and had started the recovery process. With this type of illness recovery is slow and, at times, there can be some unexplained setbacks. Knowledge is vital because the more one learns about the illness, the greater chance there is of avoiding set-backs.

Since returning from Southampton I have spent many months reading everything I can find on food and chemical allergies. I have corresponded with people throughout Australia and New Zealand who have suffered similar problems. I have also spoken to many fellow sufferers through associations such as the Myalgic Encephalomyelitis Society and other allergy groups. From all this discussion and contact one thing has become very clear — there is relatively little information, concise enough or comprehensive enough, to allow non-medical persons to understand their allergy problems. Particularly, there is very little information on the *treatment* of complex allergy problems.

Treatment, in the main, consists of identifying and then avoiding allergenic substances. However, a multi-faceted approach, using a variety of known health techniques, will most definitely speed up the recovery process and allow a return to a better standard of health than may otherwise have been achieved.

Recent research indicates that a breakdown in the body's immune system is responsible for complex allergy conditions. This breakdown can be caused by a number of factors, such as wrong feeding during infancy, a virus or other illness, hereditary factors and environmental exposure to foods and chemicals. When the immune system breaks down the body becomes overloaded with toxins and major organs, such as the liver and the intestine, cannot cope. This is a dangerous situation for the body and, as well as the immediate symptoms, because the toxins attack a target organ, it can lead to major disease or even death.

I believe the allergy problem is just beginning. Already doctors such as Julian Kenyon are being overwhelmed by the large number of patients. Hundreds of doctors throughout this country are dealing with many thousands of patients who appear to have indefinable illnesses. They continue to treat symptoms and palliate overstressed nervous systems, whilst the allergenic toxins in these people run rampant and remain undiagnosed and undetected. Whilst modern mankind continues to poison his existence with chemicals, artificial additives, refined carbohydrates and junk food, more and more people will become sicker and sicker.

It is estimated that 20 per cent of the population are now suffering from allergies, in one form or another, while 20 per cent have major allergy problems. Most of these remain undiagnosed. The worst cases are often treated for the wrong causes or classified as psychological. Many general practitioners may suspect what is wrong with their patient but may not know what to do about it. The symptoms are often masked and confused, making it impossible to link them with a specific cause. Chronic catarrh can be as easily caused by a food as by a dust or pollen. A skin rash may be the result of ingestion, not contact. Regular urinary problems may be due to diet, rather than an infection. The examples are endless.

There are many people today who are going about their everyday lives in a sort of twilight zone, neither being fully sick nor truly well.

They feel tired often. They are prone to sudden changes of mood. They catch colds regularly. They often have digestive and elimination problems. They are never really well and yet never sick enough to get to the bottom of their problem. Others are chronically ill with a range of debilitating symptoms. As fast as they get over one symptom they are struck by another. Doctors are beginning to suspect the causes, but even an alert general practitioner can do little to alleviate his patient's suffering.

To a great extent, this is an illness which must be treated by the sufferer. To this end, there is a great need for the development of guidelines for self treatment. This book is an attempt to lay down these guidelines. It seeks to explain in layman's language, what an allergy is and what to do about it. It promotes the idea that the main offenders are common to most sufferers and easily eliminated. In most cases, it is not necessary to eliminate all allergens. Dispense with the main offenders and the body's immune system will be given the assistance it needs to re-assert itself. Combine this approach with the other proven health techniques, described in this book, and recovery for most will be assured.

1

ALLERGIES

What are they?

In general terms, an allergy is a disorder which is brought about when the body adversely reacts to substances normally considered harmless. A true allergy is one which evokes certain medically-recognizable responses in the body's immune system.

Whereas non-harmful substances are metabolised effectively and broken down into approximately forty essential nutrients, allergenic substances are not. They clog the bloodstream and lymph system and are absorbed by the tissues, where they can continue to accumulate until ingestion of allergens ceases. Even then it will be days, weeks or even months, before this accumulated toxic matter is slowly dispersed by the overworked kidneys and liver.

In recent years, it has become evident that there are other types of sensitivities particularly relating to food and chemicals, which whilst not allergies in the true medical sense, are just as devastating in their effect on the body and the life of the sufferer. How the mechanisms of these sensitivities work is not fully clear. For our purposes the term allergy will be used in its broadest sense, to cover all types of adverse reactions by the body, to various substances, known as allergens.

Causes

These will be dealt with in more detail in later chapters. However, in general terms, there appear to be two categories of allergy illness. Firstly, there is the specific allergy, caused by a partially digested food substance entering the bloodstream through the intestine and causing a toxic, chemical reaction. Normally, when a food substance enters the bloodstream, enzymes and white cells in the blood, complete the digestive process. However, in an allergic person the immune system does not respond normally. It is now known that damage to the small intestine, caused by incorrect feeding as an infant, is one major cause of this. Metabolic and digestive disturbances, resulting from severe illness and genetic defects are others.

Secondly, it has become increasingly evident that in recent years, people are developing a wide range of multiple sensitivities which appear to be caused by the accumulated toxic overload of our twentieth century, Western lifestyle. Over the past thirty years, the human body has been subjected to processed foods, together with their chemical additives, in ever-increasing quantities. Combine this with chemicals from other sources, which are polluting both atmosphere and soil, and we have an increasing toxic situation in the body which is making a lot of people sick. Unfortunately, this form of illness is difficult to diagnose, and will remain so until more doctors begin to take an interest in clinical ecology; a branch of medicine which has evolved in America to deal with illness caused by the individual's environment.

Symptoms

If you suffer from any of the following medical problems on a recurring basis, you may well have an allergy to one or perhaps several substances in your diet and environment — headaches, colds, catarrh, sinusitis, hay fever, aching, skin rashes, overheating, irritated bowel, constipation, urinary infections, joint and back pain, excessive sweating, indigestion, flatulence, asthma, accelerated heartbeat, blurred vision, tight facial muscles, slurred or awkward speech and many others.

Other more general symptoms but equally as important as indicators of allergic reactions are: tiredness, depression, loss of concentration, florid face, memory difficulties, insomnia, heaviness or dullness, rheumatism, arthritis, abdominal swelling, cold feeling and many others. Many people have been going to their doctors for years and complaining of one or several of these symptoms. Time and time again, nothing further has been done for them, except a prescription for a palliative drug.

A classic example of a symptom which has been causing doctors to scratch their heads for years, is the migraine headache. Recently, London's Institute of Child Health tested eighty-eight children with severe migraine headaches. Each was placed on a special diet designed to avoid as many allergy-inducing foods as possible. The result was that eighty-two children, 93 per cent, were completely free of headache while on the diet. Foods were than reintroduced, one at a time, and all eighty-two relapsed. Finally, when the offending foods were sorted out, it was found that seventeen were allergic to one food only, while the remaining sixty-five were allergic to several foods. The most common of these were: cows' milk, eggs, chocolate, oranges and wheat, followed by cheese, tomatoes, fish, beef and pork. It was also found that the children were usually very fond of the provoking food.

Masked allergies and addiction

Dr William Philpott, one of the world leaders in the understanding of allergy related illness associates allergy conditions with the addictive process. In *Brain Allergies: The Psychonutrient Connection* which he wrote with Dr Dwight K. Kalita, (published by Keats Publishing, Inc.), Dr Philpott says:

One can say that allergy and its counterpart, addiction, along with nutritional deficiency and infection are the building blocks from which chronic diseases are built. It matters not with which one of these we start; the others will soon follow. Of these three, the most important beginning point of many illnesses, as far as our clinical evidence reveals, is that of allergy-addiction, with nutritional deficiency and infection following closely.

It is possible to eat a certain food every day, with no apparent problems and still be allergic to it. Instead of something obvious like coffee, it can be a food as innocent as eggs, wheat or chicken. Allergists refer to this situation as an 'addictive' or 'masked' allergy.

3

If you crave a particular food, and also suffer from recurring symptoms such as aching or abdominal swelling, it is most likely that you are allergic to it. The craving is often the only way of identifying the allergenic food, because the symptoms do not always occur immediately after eating the food or even in the same day.

In his book, *Dr Mandell's Five Day Allergy Relief System,* Dr Marshall Mandell found that the addictive form of allergy can go undetected.

Unlike the better known forms of food allergy from which hives, coughing, itching, facial swelling, sneezing, nasal drip, nausea, vomiting, cramps or headaches result almost at once, the addictive form of allergy is much more subtle and is rarely suspected by its victims.

Instead of having an immediate adverse reaction to the offending food, the addicted person experiences a positive feeling. It's just like the relief a heroin addict feels. We do not yet fully understand why an addictive form of food allergy exists, but we know it does!

As a result of addictive food allergies, many people suffer the effects of compulsive eating and drinking. The sufferers struggle through life, subjected to the agonies of their cravings and the instability of their moods. They do not understand what controls them and neither do their family or friends and the affect on their personal and family life can be devastating. Often they develop feelings of low self-esteem due to their inability to cope with the physical, mental and emotional disorders forced on them by the abnormal chemical reactions taking place in their bodies.

Compulsive eating

Compulsive eating is caused by one or several masked food allergies, which are invariably addictive, without the individual realizing it. Not all compulsive eaters are obese, but some reflect this condition. Others are likely to suffer from some form of overweight due to fluid retention. This is caused by the allergic response in the capillary blood vessels, when fluid passes through the capillary walls into surrounding tissues. Another cause is the build up of toxin-impregnated body fat due to inefficient metabolism that is a result of the allergic response.

A compulsive eater, plagued by an undetected, addictive allergy condition, perhaps from several foods at the same time is probably experiencing some of the following:

—Inability to miss a meal without getting a headache, fatigue or marked irritability. Once you have eaten, these discomforts miraculously disappear.

—Necessity to eat a specific food every single day, for example at the evening meal.

—Tendency to 'binge-eat' a particular food. Once you have started you cannot stop until you are almost sick, or too full to eat any more.

—A constant craving for sweets, so that you keep a supply around at all times.

—A habit of using a large amount of your favourite condiment at every meal. No meal feels complete without it.

—A need to eat wheat products, such as bread, cake, pies, spaghetti, biscuits, every day with lunch and dinner; or a craving to snack on these foods between meals and later in the evening.

—A habit of waking in the middle of the night for a piece of your favourite food before going back to sleep.

—A need to eat a large helping of ice cream, or drink a large glass of milk, before feeling relaxed enough to go to bed and sleep.

—A feeling that you could not live without your favourite food, and as a result you find it impossible to stay on a diet.

These are some of the habits exhibited by compulsive eaters who are unknowingly caught up in a vicious roundabout of craving and addiction, caused by masked food allergies.

For fifteen years I experienced most of these symptoms. When I was tired, which was most of the time, I could not cram my favourite foods into my mouth quickly enough. As soon as the first morsel of bread or drop of milk, reached my taste buds the craving intensified. Whereas a normal person would drink a glass of milk with a biscuit, I would need two or three glasses with four or five biscuits and still I would not feel satisfied. With hindsight I realize that this response was unnatural, but at the time I knew nothing about addictive allergies, and I was used to simply *liking* milk, biscuits, bread, etc. Because my diet appeared to be normal and healthy, I did not associate my predilection for certain foods with the miserable way I had been feeling for years.

The problem with this type of addiction is that withdrawal symptoms are always experienced after eating an allergenic food, once the beneficial effects have worn off. This may be after several hours, and can range from slight fatigue to severe anxiety, migraine headaches, depression, anger, exhaustion, arthritis, itching, asthma and painful muscle aching. This sets up a craving which requires a further meal or snack of the addicted food to quell the symptoms and the whole process begins again.

The solution is firstly to recognize the problem and then eliminate the offending foods from the diet. Once this happens, recurring symptoms miraculously disappear and an overloaded, toxin-laden body is replaced by a body that feels lighter, revitalized and filled with energy.

It is often difficult for relatives and friends to appreciate the severity of a chronic food-chemical allergy condition. The victim may look quite well but looks and bodily appearance can belie the chemical turmoil and damage within. The fact that he or she complains of not feeling well, and lacks vitality, is put down to nerves, lack of character, laziness, all sorts of reasons — by even the most well-meaning people. Inevitably, the poor unfortunate is accused of being a hypochondriac. Family understanding of the condition and support to help the victims avoid substances which are poisonous to them is an essential aid to recovery.

Compulsive drinking

Many people need a drink to get through the day because they are addicted to the ingredients from which their favourite alcoholic beverage is made. Consequently it seems that alcoholism and food addiction are closely related, if not identical.

Researchers at the Deaconess Hospital in St Louis, Missouri, have recently conducted an intensive enquiry into alcoholism and its possible causes. They found evidence to substantiate the belief that alcoholism is, in fact, a food allergy. Their research showed that alcoholics are twice as susceptible to food allergies as are non-drinkers. Different alcoholics were found to be addicted to the different elements within the drink, rather than alcohol itself.

Alcoholic beverages are made by fermenting sugars derived from the starches of various grains and vegetables. For example, beer contains barley and hops; whisky, malted barley; vodka, potatoes, rye or barley; wine, grapes; and so on. All alcoholic drinks contain yeast, another common allergen.

The presence of alcohol in the system acts as a catalyst to the absorption of materials from the intestinal tract. As the alcohol is absorbed, it takes along with it particles of the food from which the particular alcoholic drink was made. In addition, because of the catalystic effect of the alcohol, accelerated absorption of any drugs or foods ingested with the alcohol, also occurs.

The ingredients which make up an alcoholic beverage can produce an addictive form of food allergy which, because of the effects of the alcohol, is even more acute than food allergies without alcohol. As a result a person with this problem becomes a compulsive drinker, or to use that grossly inaccurate term — 'alcoholic'.

The chemical effect of the alcohol causes compulsive drinkers to have withdrawal symptoms that are even more intense than other food allergies. The addicted drinker, in desperation, reaches for another drink to seek relief and so perpetuates an endless cycle of ingestion and withdrawal. Dr Mandell writes about the addiction to alcohol as a food allergy.

Alcoholics may think they are drinking to combat an anxious or depressed state of mind due to some emotional problem — and a drink certainly makes them feel better fast — but, in reality, they are suffering from the addictive form of food allergy, and their anxiety and depression are nervous system allergic reactions to the food residues of the source materials in the alcoholic beverage.

As in most food-related allergies, there is an addictive process which requires larger doses more frequently, to control withdrawal symptoms and to briefly regain the feeling of well-being. This is

7

particularly so with the compulsive drinker who is locked into a cycle of withdrawal symptoms and relief, followed by recurring symptoms, which are only relieved by further alcohol. It is only when this endless cycle is permanently broken that the sufferer can regain good health. After this, abstinence is usually the only answer, although if the allergy is to grains and the person has been a beer drinker, then a change to a non grain-based drink, such as wine, may solve the problem. However, this should only be done after a period of total abstinence for at least six months, to allow the overloaded immune system to recover its full function.

People who are reliant on alcohol have often had a severe masked allergy problem from infancy. Throughout their childhood years and into their late teens, they were never well — suffering various recurring ailments, tiredness and the awful fits of depression which go with such an insidious condition. Then with their first drink of beer, or spirits, they feel much better. Others may have an initial negative reaction, followed by a beneficial feeling. The result in either case, is that the individual forms a firm attachment to the alcoholic beverage and thereafter incorporates it in his every-day life. A downward spiral commences, which may last many years, before that person reaches a stage where the alcohol will no longer relieve the symptoms no matter how much is consumed.

Most alcoholic drinks other than wine, are grain based, with wheat being a major ingredient. Therefore a close link would appear to exist between an individual's liking for foods such as bread, pies and biscuits, and a need to drink beer in excessive quantities.

Symptoms of food and chemical allergies

Central nervous system

Poor concentration
Confusion
Angry outbursts
Depression
Anxiety
Hyperactivity
Delusions
Personality changes

Fits
Dizziness
Sleeplessness
Impaired learning ability
Impaired brain activity
Lethargy
Fatigue
Drowsiness

8

Detached or withdrawn
  feeling
Poor memory
Headaches

Hallucinations
Hot flushes

Heart and blood vessels
Swelling
Palpitations
Chest pain
Inflammation of veins and
  arteries

Extra heart-beats
Angina
Varicose veins
Atherosclerosis
Rapid heart-beat

Blood
Decreased immunity to illness
Increased clotting
Decreased clotting
Anaemia (reduction in red
  cells)

Leukopenia (reduction in
  white cells)
Thrombocytopenia
Thrombosis

Eyes
Blurred vision
Itching or burning
Heavy-lidded feeling
Reading difficulties

Soreness
Sensitivity to light
Double vision

Skin
Urticaria (Hives)
Abnormal pallor
Itching
Excessive perspiration

Dryness
Eczema
Acne and pimples
Skin lesions

Muscles and joints
Muscle weakness
Muscle spasms
Muscle cramps
Muscle inflammation
  (Myositis)
Muscle stiffness

Swollen joints
Stiff joints
Aching joints
Inflammation of joints
  (Arthritis)

Stomach and intestines
Reduced appetite
Increased appetite
Abdominal pain (Colitis)
Diarrhoea
Constipation
Diverticulitis
Bloated feeling

Irritated anus
Hyperacidity
Abdominal cramps
Nausea and/or vomiting
Wind
Excessive belching
Ulcers

Urinal and genital tracts
Bladder infections
Prostatitis
Burning or painful urination
Heavy periods
Irregular periods
Painful periods

Increased sexual drive
Decreased sexual drive
Frequent urination
Bed wetting
Need to urinate during the
    night

Noses and sinuses
Blocked nose
Catarrh
Sinus infection
Reduced sense of smell

Increased sense of smell
Sneezing
Itchy nose

Ears
Ringing and buzzing noises
    (Tinnitus)
Hearing loss
Sensitivity to noise

Blocked eustachian tubes
Itching
Earache
Ear infections

Mouth and throat
Swollen throat
Throat infections
Bad taste
Hoarseness
Sore throat

Mouth ulcers
Swollen gums
Dry mouth
Overproduction of saliva

Lungs

Bad breath
Asthma
Frequent colds and flu
Chest infections
Breathing difficulties

Coughing
Hyperventilation (rapid breathing)
Hypoventilation (slow breathing)

ECOLOGICAL ILLNESS

Your environment can make you sick

Intolerant reactions to normal substances are not allergies in the true medical sense, yet they have the same symptoms and cause the same distressing health problems.

It is not yet fully understood why people become sensitive to various foods and chemicals. One theory is that the body may lack the particular enzyme necessary to digest a certain food. This may be temporary or permanent, acquired or inherited. An example of this is milk intolerance caused by a lack of lactase, the enzyme needed to digest lactose, the natural sugar in milk.

According to Drs Kenyon and Lewith of the Centre for Alternative Therapies, Southampton, 'Ecological illness is best defined as illness caused wholly or partially by food and/or chemical sensitivity. In the real sense of the word ecological illness is not strictly allergic, as the normally accepted serological accompaniments of allergic illness are not invariably present.'

Causes of ecological illness

What causes the body to become sensitive to many different foods and chemicals? At this stage the causes are not clearly understood. However the alarming number of people who are now suffering from this problem, in varying degrees, indicates that it is widespread due to the following reasons:

The excessive consumption of refined, pre-packed, tinned, frozen and artificially-preserved foods, in our Western civilization. The over-consumption of refined carbohydrates and the almost daily intake of 'fast foods', are aggravating factors.

Increasing pollution of the environment with chemicals such as fertilizers, insecticides and hydrocarbons.

The vast array of drugs and medication being prescribed daily by doctors for every conceivable complaint.

These factors are related to Western lifestyles. Many studies have shown that the tribespeople of Africa and the rural peasants of Asia, do not suffer from ecological illness. Freedom from chemicals and drugs, along with their diet of unrefined unprocessed foods, allows their immune systems to work at full potency. The result is relative freedom from allergies, cancers and heart disease.

While the individual might find it difficult to do much about the overuse of fertilizers and insecticides, it is possible to cut back on drugs and the wrong type of foods. Ecological illness, whilst being debilitating and depressing, can be overcome by personal discipline and sound management.

According to Dr Richard Mackarness in his book *Chemical Victims,* in terms of clinical ecology, the body is like a water barrel. Environmental exposure to allergens, in the form of food and chemical substances, is seen as the water. If we have an excess of environmental exposure (water), the barrel overflows and the body becomes overloaded with toxins. Once the excess exposure to allergens can be avoided, the water ceases to overflow the barrel, and the body's immune system can regain control. Symptoms then disappear and the individual returns to normal good health. Therefore it is not necessary to eliminate all allergens. Provided enough of them are eliminated, the body will again take over and deal with the remainder itself.

Symptoms — the masked allergy

These differ from the conventional allergy as they are frequently exhibited in a masked form. For this reason, clinical ecology has

13

been slow in gaining medical acceptance. However, these days the doctor specialising as a clinical ecologist, is gaining recognition in Europe and the United States. Speaking on the situation in Australia, Professor Ian Lewis of the University of Tasmania, says that the current medical training is not geared towards producing doctors that can solve problems. He feels that doctors should be taught to consider alternatives to drug therapy, rather than be overcrammed with factual knowledge. This may lead, in time, to a resumption in use of the physician's greatest historical tool — a thorough investigation of the patient's diet and environment.*

In effect, ecological illness is one large allergy. Most people today have it, to varying degrees. Within this general malaise, more specific allergies or sensitivities occur. Invariably however, exposure to the allergen does not produce an immediate or detectable response. Symptoms tend to be masked and therefore very difficult to trace back to a specific cause. For this reason most doctors are not able to diagnose a food or chemical sensitivity occurring as a masked allergy. Their lack of training, understanding and interest in this area compounds the difficulty in obtaining a correct diagnosis. Time and time again masked allergy symptoms are diagnosed as something quite different. The symptom is then treated by the doctor and the cause remains undetected. This approach will quieten the symptom for a while but it will continue to flare up regularly until the individual is classified as a chronic sufferer. The sufferer is then often placed on a prescription drug, on a semi-permanent basis, and told to live with it. Meanwhile, the allergy remains undetected, and the build-up in toxins causes further suffering and damage to an already weakened system. In the words of Drs Kenyon and Lewith —

Masked allergy may exhibit itself by a patient being exposed to a common food such as wheat, daily. No clear reactions to the wheat are shown in the patient's symptoms; for instance the patient does not exhibit an acute asthmatic wheeze after eating a slice of bread, or urticaria after eating biscuits. But a symptom

* Dr Colin Little of Bethseda Hospital, Melbourne, has used this process with considerable success, in the treatment of food and chemical intolerances.

complex which may involve asthma, accompanied by general malaise and depression, or osteoarthritis accompanied by headaches, may be the presenting complaints. The patient avoids wheat for a period of five days then, if the wheat is the major allergen, the symptoms will usually disappear. Re-exposure after this period of time will often induce an acute recurrence of the symptoms. This recurrence may occur immediately or twenty-four hours after re-exposure.

It is easy to see why masked allergies and symptoms continue to baffle the modern doctor. It would not be an exaggeration to claim that many doctors do not understand this process and, as a result, many of their patients are being treated for asthma, skin problems, lethargy, irritability, digestive problems and a whole range of symptoms whilst the real cause, the masked allergy, goes undetected.

Allergy and addiction

The clinical ecologist has long since realized that a masked food allergy is often accompanied by an addiction to that food. People who tend to eat a lot of a particular food, and suffer cravings when it is withdrawn from their diet, need look no further for the cause of their malaise. For example the severe asthmatic who may have a masked sensitivity to wheat, will often be found snacking on a piece of bread or a sandwich, because he gets a 'lift' after eating it. The asthmatic craves wheat and for a time, sometimes years, will feel better after eating it, but is never completely well or in a normal healthy state.

As time goes on that person will require more and more wheat to suppress the symptoms, and may find that the beneficial feeling the wheat provides will only last for an hour or two, followed by more symptoms. Finally, the immune system becomes exhausted and the symptoms become overriding, no matter how much bread or other wheat products are eaten. The process is similar to other forms of addiction, caused by cigarettes, drugs and alcohol.

The diagram from Dr Mackarness' book, *Chemical Victims* illustrates by stages, the addictive process of the severely allergic person. This process may span a few months or many years. During this time, the individual's health is slowly declining and he exists,

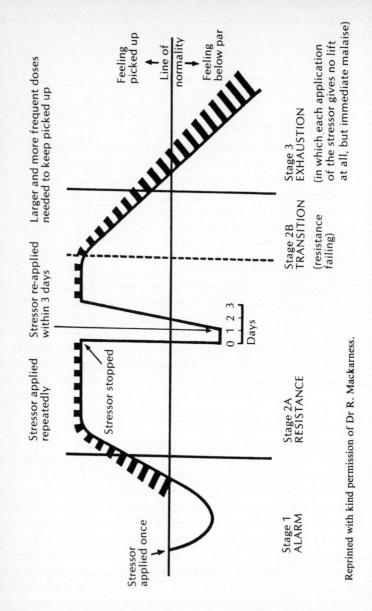

Reprinted with kind permission of Dr R. Mackarness.

16

through periods of ever-increasing illness, to a final state of chronic ill health.

The main problem is that the addictive form of food allergy is rarely suspected by its victims. In my own case, I spent many years getting sicker and sicker without realizing what was happening. People unfortunately get caught up in this situation and, after receiving no help from their doctors, tend to accept their symptoms and try to live with them instead of continuing to look for the cause.

The role of the clinical ecologist is to unmask the addiction, identify the allergenic food, or substance, and ensure its removal from the person's diet. However, as there are very few clinical ecologists, it may be necessary for the individual to carry out this process himself. This is not nearly as formidable a task as it may at first sound and is covered fully in Chapters 11 and 12.

Once the allergic food is identified it must be totally avoided, in all its forms, for a period of six months and in extreme cases, much longer. After this time has elapsed, the allergy usually disappears and the person is no longer intolerant to the allergen. Eventually however, intolerance may reappear if the food is eaten too often, especially on a daily basis. If this begins to happen, complete abstention at the outset can quickly return the individual to a normal state of tolerance. Even after tolerance has been achieved those foods should never be eaten on a daily basis. Once or twice per week should be more the rule.

Current tolerance level

Dr Mackarness says that the body has a 'tolerance level' to toxins which is relative to the state of health at the time. If the 'total body load' exceeds the 'current tolerance level' then the body will become ill and remain ill until this situation is reversed.

Sufferers of food and chemical allergies will always have a 'total body load', or TBL, which is in excess of their 'current tolerance level' or CTL. As they become progressively overloaded, their CTL continues to fall, whilst their TBL continues to increase, until the immune system is exhausted and severe illness or death results. This whole process can take many years. During this time, the victim is caught up in a continuing downhill spiral of increasing chronic ill

ALLERGY OVERLOAD

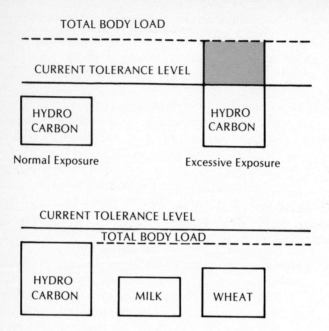

health. This situation can be halted, and finally reversed, by identifying the allergic foods and chemicals causing the overload, and removing them from diet and environment. Initially, this will require total avoidance, so that the immune system can recover and the CTL can be raised. From then on it is a matter of avoiding allergens enough, to prevent the TBL from exceeding the CTL.

The study of ecological illness in the United Kingdom, Europe and the United States, has shown that food and chemical sensitivities are often multiple. This can make diagnosis complex and difficult. Most doctors are not generally conversant with the concept that ecological illness can produce allergies with non-specific symptoms. A wide range of recurring symptoms, resulting in serious general malaise is often misunderstood.

There seems little doubt that multiple allergies, due to ecological intolerance, present a fast growing problem which could take on mammoth proportions by the end of the century.

THE IMMUNE SYSTEM

How does it work?

Irrespective of whether an allergy is classifiable in the narrow medical sense or the broader ecological sense, it is, nevertheless, a trauma, which involves a breakdown in the body's immune system.

I have found from my own experience, that a basic understanding of the immune system, how it functions and what happens to it, is an important aid in developing the correct approach to food and chemical allergies. Many of us have only the vaguest notion of how our bodies work because our education system is fundamentally barren on this subject. Also there is much about the immune system that is not yet understood. Until recently, medical science has had a narrow picture of the manner in which an allergen reacts within the body, and the resultant destructive effects. It has now been accepted that there are many other types of allergic responses which do not fit into the understood pattern. However, for this brief look at the immune system, it suffices to use the conventional medical interpretation of an allergic reaction.

The purpose of the immune system is to guard the body against viruses, germs, undigested protein and any other substances which are likely to be harmful or toxic. These substances are known collectively, as antigens. One of the first signs of failure in the immune system, is a growing tendency to suffer from colds and 'flu. As a result, further weakening of the immune system may exacerbate a susceptibility to food and chemical sensitivities.

The immune response

The first phase of the immune response occurs when antigens enter the body, usually through the mouth, nose or skin. When this happens, inflammation occurs in the body and the immune system is stimulated to produce more white cells. The task of these extra white cells is to eliminate the offending antigen. If this is successful, the inflammation will subside.

The same process will apply when the body is stressed emotionally or physically. Further stress on the immune system can be caused by an allergic reaction due to the presence in the body of antigens, in the form of allergenic substances.

The second phase of the immune response takes place when the white cells (called leucocytes) are unable to destroy the antigen. The immune system then commences the formation of antibodies, called immunoglobulins, which are tailor-made to combat the antigen and destroy it. Once antibodies have been created to fight a specific antigen, they remain dormant in the body, ready for any future invasion by the antigen. The body now has the capacity to produce more of that antibody, faster, the next time invasion takes place. This is the principle used in immunization and is called Specific Immunity.

Thus, there are two stages to an immune response. The first being, the production of white cells, and the second being, the creation of specific antibodies. Normally, the white cells and the antibodies destroy the antigen and the body makes a speedy recovery. Sometimes however, this does not happen and the result is an allergic reaction which the immune system cannot deal with.

The allergic reaction

There are five different classes of immunoglobulins in the body. These are known as IgG, IgA, IgM, IgD and IgE. IgG is the principal immunoglobulin in the blood and internal fluids. Its job is to remove soluble antigens from the body, in conjunction with other immune complexes. IgA, and to a lesser extent IgM are the main secretory immunoglobulins. They form a protective coating on the body's mucosa, thereby limiting entrance of antigens through the mucosa surfaces, such as in the nasal passages and the gut. Evidently, the physiological functions of IgD and IgE are not fully understood. It is thought that IgE may play an important part in ridding the body of mucosal infection but is ineffective in ecological illness. On the other hand, IgD may act as the trigger to initiate immune responses as it has been observed that, when a mucosal surface is under attack by antigens, initiation of IgE production is dependent upon a lymphocyte that contains IgD.

When the antigen is an allergenic substance (the allergen), the leucocytes and immunoglobulins are unable to cope with it. The antibody and the antigen react, causing a malfunction in the body's defences. The mast cells, which are found in mucous membrane and connective tissue, break up. As a result, chemicals such as histamine, are released and these cause irritation and damage.

Some antigens may reach the bloodstream by way of the body's mucous surfaces. There, they attach themselves to red and white cells or form immune complexes with specific antibodies. These are carried around the body and can cause direct tissue injury, for example a precipitate in connective tissue which can block small blood vessels. This results in fever, aching, muscle pains, and can happen after eating a certain food. Those mysterious, but troublesome, back and joint pains which appear to have no rational cause, can be the result of an allergic reaction. Alternatively, the symptoms may not relate to a specific 'target' area. Instead, inflammation and fever may occur over the entire body. This can make it difficult to identify as an allergic reaction.

When inflammation or fever occurs as part of the immune response, it may be localized at an area of infection or be dispersed throughout the entire body. If the latter happens, the body temperature will increase and cause greater enzyme activity. This in turn, increases the metabolic rate; providing extra energy for the production of the leucocytes and immunoglobulins needed to fight the invading antigens. Although, in the case of an allergic reaction, this process is not successful, it may explain why allergy sufferers, particularly of food and chemical allergies, often tend to feel overheated.

The blood

The ability of the immune system to fight disease is dependent upon the level of general health and physical fitness. However, even a healthy body will have its immunocompetence severely reduced by excessive stress or fatigue. The reason for this is that, amongst other things, stress increases the viscosity of the blood.

The blood is an all-important factor in the promotion of effective immune responses. A high blood viscosity brought about by stress, or lack of physical fitness, results in a breakdown of efficiency in the components of the immune system. When a person is physically unfit, overweight or stressed, the blood becomes clogged with cholesterol, triglycerides (fats), and various waste products. The fat causes the red cells to stick together with tiny particles called platelets, whose function is to clot the blood in the event of injury. As a result, the blood becomes sludgy and sticky and its oxygen-carrying capacity is reduced. This factor, plus the narrowing of arteries by cholesterol deposits, means that it can no longer flow freely.

When these circumstances occur, the white cells and antibodies cannot function properly, resulting in impairment of the immune system. It is vital therefore, in the treatment of chronic allergy conditions, to achieve and maintain low blood viscosity. This can be done by shedding excess weight, regular exercise and the reduction of dietary cholesterol and fats.

Infancy

The newborn baby does not have a fully functioning immune system or digestive system. These develop during the first twelve months of life. During this critical period, the child is dependent on the mother's milk to provide immunoglobulins for protection and enzymes for digestion. Breast milk contains substances which give the infant immunity, as well as nutrients and enzymes in the exact proportion necessary for the baby's needs. For this reason, a baby should be breast-fed for at least the first six months of life. If the child is introduced to foreign substances, such as cow's milk and cereals too early, permanent damage to the developing immune system and lifelong allergy problems can result.

During the first few months of life a child does not produce enough enzymes to break down introduced foods sufficiently. A baby's gut is very porous and relies on a secretion from the mother's breast, called colostrum, which acts as a coating, thus preventing harmful protein molecules passing through the gut wall into the blood.

If the child is denied this protection, undigested food particles will enter the bloodstream and confuse the developing immune system, which then accepts them as normal. This causes immunological havoc and instead of being digested by enzymes and white cells, the substances may be ignored by the immune system and left to cause allergy reactions. The problem may continue into adult life, causing further damage to the body and increasing illness. (See 'Enzymes' — Chapter 16).

Helping the immune system

Immunotherapy is one method of attempting to help or stimulate the immune system to overcome a disease condition. With respect to complex allergy problems, especially those concerning food and chemicals, this approach is rarely successful. Apart from the difficulty in obtaining accurate diagnosis, the process seeks to stimulate something which is often too overloaded to respond.

The most effective method of helping the immune system is by diet and exercise. Abstinence from allergenic foods, together with additional nutrients and a common sense approach to regular exercise, will cleanse the blood, reduce stored toxins and encourage the immune system to rebuild its efficiency.

4

M.E.

Myalgic encephalomyelitis — The multi-allergy menace

Myalgic encephalomyelitis, commonly known as M.E., is an ongoing condition, resulting from a severe viral or other illness. Another name for this condition is post viral syndrome. It is not in itself infectious but occurs when the victim is left with a damaged immune system, causing a range of debilitating symptoms. They include, extreme tiredness, aching, muscle weakness and impairment of some mental processes.

Symptoms, such as these, are not uncommon after viral infections, but rarely persist for more than a few weeks and then do not recur. However, when they do persist, or regularly recur for an abnormal period of time, perhaps for more than a year, then an ongoing illness emerges which is totally different to the original illness. In addition to a range of chronic and persistent symptoms, the victim also develops a masked intolerance to many foods, chemicals and inhalants. Life becomes very unpleasant indeed. The sufferers do not understand what is happening to them and usually neither do their doctors. Many doctors refuse to acknowledge the existence of multiple allergies or the illnesses that cause them. They continue to treat the symptoms, while ignoring a mass of evidence as to their cause, which has been readily available for more than a decade, particularly from the US.

Myalgic encephalomyelitis has been known by many other names over the past thirty years and has been reported in the *British Medical Journal* under such names as Icelandic Disease, Royal Free Disease and Akuryeri Disease, prior to its present name being commonly adopted. In America the same illness is known as neuromyasthenia. Like all illnesses involving multiple masked allergies, the most important factor in finding effective treatment is an awareness, by doctor and patient, that such illnesses exist, and are responsible for a wide range of chronic symptoms. There is still a long way to go before this awareness reaches a satisfactory level in this country.

During the past three years, there has been a number of reported outbreaks in Australia and New Zealand. Evidently the illness has a history of localized epidemicity with outbreaks being reported in institutional situations such as large hospitals, army barracks and schools, and thought to be due to an unidentified virus which remains in the body and causes continuing symptoms. The majority of sufferers however, appear to have been left with the condition as a result of some other serious illness which has had a damaging effect on the immune system.

In recent years, myalgic encephalomyelitis has become such an increasing problem in Western countries that M.E. Societies have been formed to help people cope with the illness, and to encourage medical research into its causes. There is still very little known about it and if it were not for the efforts of Professor Stewart Goodwin, of the Royal Perth Hospital, and one or two others, M. E. sufferers would continue to grow ill without adequate medical help.

M.E. has not been reported in Third World countries. This probably indicates that the breakdown in our natural resistance to disease, caused by the chemicals in our over-refined Western diet, is making us very susceptible to illness. Particularly to illnesses which leave the victim with a damaged immune system. Often, the result is a multiple allergy condition with a wide range of symptoms, not commonly attributable to allergies. Due to the masked nature of the symptoms, the sufferer is left puzzled and perplexed.

It must be stressed that M.E. is a particular disease which incorporates multiple allergy symptoms, usually in a masked form. There are many other causes of chronic allergy illness, and this book seeks to provide a general insight into as many of them as possible.

What does myalgic encephalomyelitis mean?

According to Dr R. Loblay, who is senior lecturer in immunology at Sydney University: 'The term itself means an inflammatory condition of the brain and spinal cord and in retrospect is an unsatisfactory name for the condition. It was coined not long after the 1955 epidemic at the Royal Free Hospital in London, at a time when poliomyelitis was at its peak, and the outbreak was at first feared to be polio.' Dr Loblay goes on to say that extensive tests have never shown evidence of an inflammatory process in the brain or spinal cord. Invariably the blood count and ESR (indication of inflammation) are normal, which indicates that some other type of pathological process is going on which is non-inflammatory.

In the past Dr Loblay says the medical profession has been reluctant to accept M.E. as a bona fide illness because of this lack of laboratory evidence. However doctors are beginning to realize that they cannot continue to ignore the illness. Based on Dr R.W. Gorringe's estimates in New Zealand, there could be well over 50,000 people suffering from M.E. in Australia; mostly undiagnosed. It appears that M.E. has become another manifestation of the over-chemicalised, twentieth century lifestyle.

Symptoms

The most dominant symptoms are persistent exhaustion, muscle weakness and impaired mental function. In some cases the disease can progress to a point where bed rest for a prolonged period is required. Because this is a polysymptomatic illness, the sufferer is rarely free of symptoms. It seems that all parts of the body are affected at various times with a constantly changing symptomatology. Often three or four symptoms are raging at the same time. Some sufferers will experience headaches, blurred vision, hearing loss, stiff and aching muscles, facial and neck stiffness, overheating, white pallor, inflamed red pallor, extreme fatigue, extreme nervous tension, sleeplessness, constant colds, urinary infections, constipation, digestive problems, bloatedness and aching back. Others may suffer from memory loss, poor concentration, cold hands and feet, irritable outbursts, moodiness, depression, heavy sweating, proneness to drop things, difficulty in finding the right words, tinnitus and apathy. These symptoms are all continuously aggravated by the individual's ignorance of the fact that he will have developed masked allergies to some, or even many foods and other substances.

Inability to recall events, to think clearly and to comprehend, are common and devastating effects of this illness. They are also among the most tragic, as they affect the very core of one's existence. This problem is further exacerbated by stress. Memory blackouts and confusion can occur at the most inappropriate moment, often causing further problems. Anger, frustration, extreme irritability, and depression are often associated with these events.

M.E. has many symptoms. If you have experienced recurring symptoms in only one or two of the described categories, you do not have this condition. However, you may well have one or more, masked food allergies. These should be tracked down before the continuing overload of toxins further impairs immune efficiency and damages bodily functions, perhaps permanently.

Treatment

Apart from getting as much rest as possible, interspersed with careful, moderate excercise, the major solution to overcoming M.E. symptoms is to identify the food and chemical allergies resulting from the illness. Until identified, these substances will continue to aggravate the condition and cause the repeated flare-up of symptoms. Once the allergens have been removed, the individual always improves and, in many cases, a slow recovery to good health has been achieved. Without the removal of allergens an M.E. sufferer cannot recover. Therefore, the most vital first step to recovery is the identification and removal of all food and chemical allergens from the diet and environment.

M.E. sufferers are particularly sensitive to chemicals. Even such seemingly innocuous things as perfumes, after shaves and scented soaps can bring on fatigue, aching, headaches, catarrh and dizziness within a few seconds of exposure. Hydrocarbon fumes such as petrol fumes, exhaust fumes and pressure pack sprays are particularly dangerous. Chemicals and preservatives in food and drink are another constant aggravator and must be removed from the diet. Avoidance of chemicals in food, drink and in the air, is the key to allowing an overloaded immune system to commence a long and slow recovery. This may take one or two years but improvement will invariably result if these rules are firmly followed. It is important to seek help for this problem from a medical practitioner or naturopath, who understands the illness and is prepared to spend the time necessary to help you get well. When seeking to eliminate foods that have become toxic because of M.E., there is a widespread tendency to regard 'natural foods' as healthier than those with artificial additives. This is not necessarily the case. Many additives, particularly preservatives, are chemically identical to those found naturally in food. However, concentrations in food containing artificial additives, can be much higher than those found naturally. When these are ingested reguarly from a variety of processed foods, they can overload the system and cause allergy illness.

Because M.E. intolerances are essentially chemically caused, whether by direct exposure, or through food and other substances, many foods that contain these chemicals, in natural form, can cause further illness to M.E. sufferers. Examples are those foods containing salicylates and benzoates in comparatively high amounts, and these can be some of the seemingly innocuous fruits and vegetables. It is essential therefore, to suspect all foods, until a process of testing (described in a later chapter) can safely eliminate those that are doing harm. Merely changing one's diet to whole grains, nuts, yoghurt, fruit and vegetables, etc. will not be successful and can, if anything, worsen both disease and symptoms.

It is absolutely essential for all M.E. sufferers to take a complete range of supplementary nutrients to assist their recovery. Without supplementation of vitamins, minerals, trace elements, amino acids and most important of all, enzymes, any attempts to recover will be a waste of time. More detail is given to this subject in Chapter 15.

Exercise is important during the recovery phase to stimulate metabolism, particularly to switch back on currently inoperative oxygenase enzymes. However, it must not be overdone. Because M.E. sufferers take four times as long as healthy persons to recover from exercise, it should be commenced at about one quarter capacity and built up very slowly. It is a mistake to do more than this. Ability to recover from exercise must be almost immediate. If taken beyond this point, more harm than good will be done and a relapse will surely occur. For further information on exercise, see Chapter 19.

Because of the nature of some the symptoms of M.E. many doctors label the sufferer as 'psychologically unsound'. Fortunately, there are a few doctors throughout the country who take this illness seriously, and they are to be found by contacting the State branch of the M.E. Society.

What causes M.E.?

Dr Janice Bishop, writing in the *Medical Journal of Australia,* describes M.E. as:

> The preferred descriptive name for a poorly defined syndrome with a possible variety of causes (of which an antecedent viral infection is the most likely), which occurs sporadically and in epidemics, and results in a prolonged, frequently relapsing disorder characterised by a peculiar muscle weakness, severe head, neck and limb pains, mental changes and a varying incidence of symptoms and objective neurological findings in the central, peripheral and autonomic nervous systems. The central and dominant feature is abnormal muscle fatigue, which often has a diurnal periodicity.

She points out that during the past fifty years, since the first epidemic was reported in Los Angeles in 1934, approximately thirty epidemics have been reported in Britain, USA, Iceland, Switzerland, Alaska, Australia, Denmark, Europe and South Africa.

Dr A.M. Ramsay, honorary consultant physician to the Royal Free Hospital, London, in an article published in the *British Medical Journal,* says:

> In recent years routine antibody tests on patients suffering from myalgic encephalomyelitis have shown raised titres to Coxsackie Group B viruses. It is fully established that these viruses are the aetiological agents (the cause) of Epidemic Myalgia or Bornholm Disease and together with Echo viruses, they comprise the commonest known virus invaders of the central nervous system.

This must not be taken to imply that Coxsackie viruses are the sole agents of myalgic encephalomyelitis since any generalised virus infection may be followed by a period of post viral debility. Indeed the particular invading microbial agent is probably not the most important factor. Recent work suggests that the key to the problem is likely to be found in the abnormal immunological response of the patient to the organism.

Dr David Smith, medical adviser to the M.E. Society of Great Britain, describes M.E. as a 'post viral syndrome'.

It is quite clear from the studies that this particular syndrome, this complex of symptoms, is related to many viruses. It is often Coxsackie B virus which is responsible but it can also be the Echo viruses or Epstein-Barr viruses; post jaundice syndrome and in one case, a chicken pox virus. It is therefore unimportant what name is given M.E. We are still presented with a group of people suffering from a complex post viral syndrome, a complex of undisputed suffering and problems.

These extracts show that informed, senior medical practitioners, who have studied the disease, are in agreement that M.E. originates from a viral infection which affects the cells and damages the immune system. The most debilitating after-effect is the inability of the body to cope with a wide range of foods and chemicals, as well as airborne allergens. This multiple allergy condition is responsible for the multitude of symptoms which constantly plague the sufferer. Once the intolerances are removed, the immune system ceases to be overloaded and the body's natural mechanisms can begin to repair the damage.

The leading authority on M.E. in New Zealand, Dr R.W. Gorringe, suggests that the immune system of the M.E. sufferer is already abnormal to start with. He goes on to say:

The long-term effect on health is more insidious than first imagined and should not be seen just in simplistic pharmacological terms such as blood levels, excretion rates and so on, but rather attention needs to be directed towards the whole individual and their sense of well-being, level of energy, ability to think and concentrate, initiative, drive, spontaneity, quality of sleep and inter-personal relationship changes.

Dr Gorringe reports that he, personally, looks after one hundred M.E. cases within his practice, and his contacts with other doctors in New Zealand, indicates that there would be at least a further 10,000 sufferers in that country. However, he concedes that most of these people are not recognized as such by their doctors.

M.E. as a clinical syndrome is a multi-systems disease. There are at least sixty-four possible symptoms that can be present in part, or all, at any one time. It is probably this more than anything, that has caused doctors and other people to find difficulty in grasping the reality of M.E. The problem is that doctors are taught to believe in the law of parsimony. This attempts to ascribe a single cause to a single problem, and doctors are taught to look for the lesion or the problem to explain a set of circumstances or symptoms. If multiple symptoms are presented involving multiple systems of the body and which apparently lack cohesive features or a common thread, then this model breaks down. It is then the next most common mistake to use a psychological model and say therefore this is a psychological problem. The commonest labels that people get put on them are 'neurotic', 'hypochondriac' and 'depressed'. As blanket diagnoses these are cruelly untrue and a cop-out.

In his excellent book *Brain Allergies: the Psychonutrient Connection* Dr Philpott recognizes this problem and outlines the correct approach for doctors:

To consider all these apparently different states in terms of a simple disease process provides a valuable framework for treatment, whether the presenting symptomatology be mental or physical. Treating the basic underlying disease process rationally offers a much better prospect of achieving a final and lasting success than does the use of traditional methods.

Dr Gorringe says that people who have M.E. will inevitably develop multiple food and chemical allergies, leading to worsening metabolic malfunction. The affects of this on the mental processes of the sufferer cannot be overstated. The neuro-transmitters in the brain are affected, resulting in incomplete thought processes. This can happen often, but irregularly and particularly in times of stress.

The effects on the life of the sufferer can be devastating. Dr Philpott provides an in-depth explanation as to how and why these mental changes take place and anyone with these problems, should study his book thoroughly.

Myalgic encephalomyelitis is a residual condition, caused by another illness, in most cases a viral infection. It leaves the individual in a state of chronic ill health with a wide range of perplexing and distressing symptoms. These are perpetuated by the continuing toxic effects of food and chemical intolerances, caused by the disease. Once these allergies or intolerances are identified and removed, the toxic overload in the body, reduces to a point where the damaged immune system can begin to recover.

Recovery is possible, although it will sometimes be a slow and frustrating process. By applying the principles contained here in Part II, the sufferer will see a marked improvement in their condition. M.E. is simply another source of multiple allergy illness, and the rules for recovery apply equally to it, as to any other source; for example, candidiasis, coeliac disease and ecological illness.

Further benefits can be gained by the use of additional nutrients and where there is a Candida link, mycostatin can be of great benefit if taken for an extended period.

Recent studies, carried out at Otago Medical School, New Zealand, have shown that the red blood cells of M.E. sufferers are too stiff to pass easily through the capillaries. This affects blood flow to the tissues throughout the body and reduces oxygenation which in turn, causes the tissues to become inflamed and to build up extra toxins. Present indications are that daily doses of evening primrose oil will reduce the problem and may even reverse it entirely, by changing red blood cells back to normal pliability.

People wishing to know more about the illness, and where to find an informed doctor, should contact the M.E. Society in their particular State. For those battling with a current multiple allergy problem, it is important to remember that myalgic encephalomyelitis is only one of many possible causes.

5

CANDIDIASIS

The yeast allergy — an increasing problem

Amongst the wide range of substances to which people are allergic, one of the most universally common is yeast. A great number of allergy sufferers have a sensitivity to yeast in one form or another. Candida albicans is a living yeast that has been regarded as a harmless parasite, however it is now known to be the cause of candidiasis, a serious and widespread disease. Many allergists suspect that candidiasis is the root cause of multiple allergy illness. It is invariably present in some form, in cases of food and chemical allergies. Because of this, I feel strongly that this particular subject should be examined closely. Often the rectification of a yeast intolerance alone, will result in the eventual disappearance of a host of other allergies that have been plaguing the sufferer for years.

Candida albicans

Until fairly recently Candida albicans was considered to be a harmless parasite which is carried by a significant percentage of the population. It is, in effect, a living yeast which consists of minute, single cell plants or fungi. Normally, this fungus lives harmlessly inside us, along with other microbes kept in check by the immune system. But if, for some reason, the immune system is not functioning properly, or if antibiotics destroy other microbes, the Candida albicans takes advantage of this situation and spreads.

In a paper written by Dr Patricia Lucas of Germantown,

Tennessee, entitled 'Clinical Ecology Patients and Candida albicans', she writes:

> Candida albicans is a known pathogen capable of causing serious disease. Since World War Two, candidiasis has become one of the most common nosocomial, or hospital-acquired, infections. This increasing incidence is associated with the advent of antibiotics and other modern medical therapies, including immunosuppressive treatment of various diseases.

In other words, the widespread use of antibiotics and other drugs in many cases, is leading to a breakdown in the immune system. Once this happens, chronic illness sets in as the body becomes intolerant to one substance after another. Multiple food and chemical allergies develop and the individual becomes burdened by persistent, debilitating symptoms.

According to Dr Lucas, there are two main types of medically recognized candidal infection. Firstly, systemic candidiasis occurs when the yeast parasite gains entrance to the lymph system and the bloodstream, and circulates throughout the body causing infection to one or several organs. Secondly, in chronic mucocutaneous candidiasis, the yeast infects the skin and mucous membranes of the body. As the former is extremely difficult to detect, and the latter considered rare, doctors normally do not give much thought to candidiasis as something which will bear fruitful investigation.

However, what Dr Lucas and her associates have discovered, in recent years, is that a large number of people do have a form of candidiasis. They took cultures from multiple allergy patients that showed in every case that these people were carriers of Candida albicans. They then proceeded to investigate, on the basis that these patients might suffer a type of candidiasis which did not fall into the two previously recognized groups. They found that in healthy people, colonisation of the mucosa in the intestine and other places was limited by a protective coating of mucous and secreted antibodies. These two mechanisms prevented the Candida yeast from *getting in* and doing harm.

In allergy sufferers however, their findings indicated that the protective mucous coating, particularly in the small intestine, was eroded at certain points, allowing the Candida to gain entrance to the body across a resultantly 'leaky' mucosa. This damage to the intestine could have been brought about by incorrect feeding during infancy. Once Candida gains access to the bloodstream, turmoil results as the immune system, swamped by the abnormally large numbers of Candida antigens, struggles to manufacture enough antibodies to destroy them. This situation is further aggravated by the apparent involvement of a Candida immunosuppressive mechanism that renders the immune system impotent to the yeast invasion. It is thought that the cause of such immunosuppression is the heavy circulating load of candidal antigens, combined with the body's tendency to increased production of the immunosuppressive hormone, corticosterone. Thus other food and chemical substances which gain access to the bloodstream, are free to provoke allergic reactions, unhindered by the immune system.

This means that a previously undetected yeast intolerance, in the form of inapparent candidiasis, can be responsible for chronic multiple allergy illness. The good news for allergy sufferers is that this disease can be effectively treated, once diagnosed. Laboratory tests, called ELISA (Enzyme-Linked Immunosorbent Assays), have been developed in the United States to enable a more accurate diagnosis of candidiasis.

Dr C. Orian Truss of Birmingham, Alabama, is one of a number of eminent internists and allergists in the United States who has studied the Candida problem, both clinically and scientifically. In his excellent paper titled 'Restoration of Immunologic Competence to Candida albicans', published in the *Journal of Orthomolecular Psychiatry,* he refers to the 'paralysing' effect of Candida on the immune system which causes 'toxic responses to soluble yeast products'. He says that the cause of the paralysis is an overloading of yeast toxins in the system. Once this overload is reduced back to a manageable level, the immune system regains its function and can effectively deal with the problem.

Of the greatest importance to many patients with chronic candidiasis is the development of intolerance to foods, drugs and chemicals. A careful history often reveals the earliest of these intolerances occurring in the first several years after the symptoms of chronic yeast infection. Thereafter occurs a rapidly accelerating inability to tolerate environmental chemicals, whether they be as 'foods', 'drugs' or 'chemicals'. Eventually these patients may literally become unable to live in normal environments resorting for relief to the most dramatic measures of environmental control. They are unable to work and may even move to remote areas in their attempt to minimise the total load of chemicals contacted in their daily lives.

The doyen of American Allergists, Dr Theron Randolph, has since 1962, published several medical papers and articles on the connection between yeast infection and multiple masked allergy illness. According to Dr Randolph, the problem began in the 1950s, which coincides with the commencement of widespread, and often irresponsible, prescription by doctors of antibiotics, particularly broad spectrum antibiotics, which are harmful to the immune system. Dr Truss makes the point that all drugs are potentially lethal to the immune system. Prolonged exposure enables Candida to become systemic, resulting in further intolerances to drugs, foods and chemicals.

It is important to remember that each of us is different and can be affected to varying degrees. Many people have candidiasis-linked allergy problems and, as a result, may have suffered a lifetime of ill health without the cause ever becoming known.

Symptoms

An exhaustive investigation into the patient's history may uncover a pattern and range of symptoms which will lead to an accurate diagnosis of candidiasis. This procedure can be carried out by any competent medical doctor, yet it is almost impossible to find a doctor who will do this. There are signs that doctors are slowly becoming more interested in the symptoms of candidiasis. Hopefully, the result will be greater awareness of candidiasis, and of the fact that a previously unknown, systemic form of this disease is causing a lot of people chronic allergy illness.

Dr Truss in his study of this condition, links immunosuppressant drugs with the symptoms of yeast infection.

Historical examination will show the influence of birth control pills, antibiotics and cortisone and other immunosuppressant drugs. The onset of local symptoms of yeast infection in relation to the use of these drugs is especially significant and usually precedes a systemic Candida response. Repeated courses of antibiotics and birth control pills lead to ever increasing symptoms of mucosal infections in the vagina and gastrointestinal tract.

These infections are often the secondary result of inflamed mucous membranes caused by allergic responses to yeast products. Amongst the resultant symptoms are repeated infections of the respiratory tract, urethra and bladder. The normal procedure of prescribing antibiotics for these symptoms, frequently aggravates and perpetuates the underlying cause, if it is systemic candidiasis.

A classic symptom is depression, associated with difficulty in memory, reasoning and concentration. Loss of confidence and explosive irritability may follow. Evidently, endometriosis in women who have undergone hysterectomy is also common. A further complication is the development of multiple tolerances to food and chemicals, making it extremely difficult for the individual to lead a normal life. Once the yeast problem is brought under control, many, or all of the accompanying allergies disappear.

According to Dr William Crook, in his book *The Yeast Connection,* common symptoms, resulting from infection by Candida albicans (candidiasis), are as follows:

1 Feel 'bad all over' yet the cause cannot be identified and treatment of many kinds has not helped.

2 Craving for sweets.

3 Craving for other carbohydrates such as bread and pizza.

4 Sweets either make symptoms worse or give initial relief followed by worsening.

5 Craving for alcohol.

6 Bothered by persistent or recurrent athletes foot , fungus infection of the nails or 'jock itch'.

7 Feel bad on damp days or in mouldy places. Humidity also causes problems.

8   Tobacco smoke, perfumes and chemical smells make you ill.

9   Persistent and recurrent infections of the nose, throat, sinuses, ears, bronchials, bladder and kidneys.

10   Fatigue, headache or depression.

Usually these symptoms are accompanied by the following historical scenario:

1   Prolonged courses of broad-spectrum antibiotic drugs including tetracyclines, ampicillin, amoxycillin, the cephalosporins, and sulphonamides such as septra and bactrim.

2   Diet has contained a lot of yeast and sugar.

3   Signs of hypoglycaemia which tests fail to confirm.

4   History of taking birth control pills or other corticosteroid drugs.

5   Have had multiple pregnancies.

6   Recurrent problems affecting the reproductive organs such as abdominal pain, prostatitis, impotence, vaginal infection, premenstrual tension or irregularities.

Other recurring symptoms, such as tiredness, runny nose, canker sores, dizziness, nausea, frequent urination, irritability, numbness and tingling are experienced regularly and, in some cases, more or less constantly.

Treatment of chronic candidiasis.

Avoid wrong foods

For sufferers of candidiasis avoidance of carbohydrates is of prime importance. Yeasts ferment fats and proteins poorly, but thrive on carbohydrates, particularly sugars. A rigid abstinence from refined carbohydrates should be observed to prevent Candida increase in the body. The types of foods to avoid are sugars, breads, cakes and pastries etc., mushrooms, aged cheeses, dried fruits and alcoholic beverages. If possible these foods should be discarded completely on a regular basis until the candidiasis is under control. Occasional ingestion does not seem to matter but, when eaten continuously they will feed Candida albicans and constantly aggravate and worsen, a candidiasis condition. The result is ongoing allergy illness.

High protein foods, including fish, seafoods, lean meats, nuts and eggs, should take preference, combined with low carbohydrate vegetables such as lettuce, spinach, broccoli, squash, cauliflower, cucumbers and asparagus. Additional benefits may be gained by restricting cereal grains, as many people will find themselves intolerant to these because of the candidiasis. Obviously, it is not desirable to stay on a protein oriented diet for too long. However, supplementation with plenty of low carbohydrate vegetables does not only help overcome the Candida problem but will also provide an excellent diet for the maintenance of general good health.

It is important for allergy sufferers to remember to test each food before including it in a yeast free diet. Due to the candidiasis, allergies may have already developed to some of the suggested foods such as fish, nuts and eggs.

Avoid antibiotics and immunosuppressants

Antibiotics should not be taken, unless absolutely unavoidable. In particular, the 'broad-spectrum' drugs, that destroy the protective bacteria in the intestinal and vaginal tracts, should not be taken over a long term. When this is unavoidable, an antifungal drug, such as nystatin, should also be taken to counteract stimulation of yeast growth by the antibiotic.

Of particular danger is the long-term treatment of acne by the use of tetracycline. This is a common mistake made by skin specialists. One of their standard procedures is to prescribe a broad spectrum antibiotic for months at a time. Whilst this can help acne in the short term, it rarely works long term. The antibiotic causes further increase in the yeast infection which was often the root cause of the acne infection. In other words, like most skin disorders, acne is usually the sign of a deep-seated allergy disorder. Any long-term treatment by antibiotics will breakdown the immune system, promote candidiasis and result in further allergy illness.

Another condition arising from candidiasis, for which antibiotics are commonly prescribed, is urethritis. This is often diagnosed by doctors as the more serious and deeper-seated disease of cystitis of the bladder, because they do not understand candidiasis or its symptoms. As a result, antibiotics may be prescribed for weeks or even months. They do very little good and can actually harm the patient by aggravating the yeast infection which is causing the urethritis.

A further misuse of antibiotics is in their prescription for viral infections. They are not effective for this purpose, yet doctors continue to prescribe them, knowing this to be the case. General practitioners simply cannot grasp, or do not want to grasp, the simple possibility that viruses can cause infections by gaining access to the body through mucous membranes already irritated by allergic reactions to foods and chemicals. Candidiasis is considered a prime cause of this condition and antibiotics will only serve to aggravate the situation further.

Immunosuppressant drugs, such as cortisone and steroids should be avoided as they contribute to the breakdown of the immune system. These drugs will enhance the growth of yeast by their function which is designed to suppress the immune system in order to give relief of symptoms. This is a classic example of treating the symptom and not the cause. In this case the prescription of immunosuppressant drugs is actually harmful because, although in the short term symptoms will be relieved, ultimately the increased growth of yeast caused by suppressing the normal immune mechanisms will result in the deterioration of the patient's condition. More intolerances and more debilitating symptoms will then occur.

Contraceptive hormones

This is a real problem for women with candidiasis who are on the pill. It is estimated that acute vaginal candidiasis (thrush) is caused by the contraceptive pill in up to 35 per cent of women, with many other women being affected to lesser degrees. Chronic yeast vaginitis is worse during pregnancy and at certain times of the month when progesterone hormone levels are high. Therefore it is thought that the progesterone component of oral contraceptives is the cause of further aggravation of vaginal candidiasis.

A yeast infection, anywhere in the body, provides a 'reservoir' for Candida albicans, from which a systemic form of the infection can develop. The resultant breakdown in health, combined with the further development of food and chemical allergies, can be catastrophic. It is vital, therefore, to eliminate anything, be it foods or drugs, which will encourage the growth of yeast in the body. This may well mean a year or two off the pill to enable the immune system to overcome the yeast build-up and restore good health.

Avoid mouldy environments

Because candidiasis is a yeast infection, it thrives on moulds. Not only must sufferers avoid foods containing moulds, including those which are invisible to the naked eye, such as yeast in bread, mushrooms, dried fruit and cheeses, they must also avoid situations where mould spores are endemic in the atmosphere. Candidiasis sufferers will notice that when in supermarkets, they feel tired, headachy, fuzzy in the head, and can even develop breathing problems. This is partly due to the yeast spores floating around in the atmosphere from countless yeast-containing products stacked on the shelves.

Symptoms will also be aggravated where there is dampness, such as in a basement, or near poorly drained areas and bodies of water. Sneezing, running nose and aching are other immediate reactions likely in such situations. Humidity levels are another vital factor. Candidiasis sufferers will invariably feel worse when humidity is higher than usual. For this reason, avoid water-evaporative air cooling in home and office environments.

Therapy with anti-fungal drugs

There are several drugs that kill or suppress the growth of Candida albicans in the body. One of these is ketaconazole, which is a powerful drug for getting at deep-seated Candida, but should not be used long-term. Others are flagyl, nystatin and mycostatin, which are all effective antifungals capable of being used with safety for up to a year. Obviously drugs are to be avoided whenever possible. In the case of candidiasis, it has been found that long-term treatment, with an antifungal drug, is of great benefit in reducing the level of yeast in the body back to manageable proportions, which the immune system can then take over and again effectively control. However, because of the individual's previous susceptibility to Candida, continuous avoidance of all yeast-containing and yeast-encouraging foods must be maintained in order to remain permanently free of the problem. Otherwise, a recurrence is most likely.

The drug nystatin is particularly safe to the body, in general, as it is poorly absorbed through the intestinal tract. It is considered effective only for yeast infections of mucosal and skin surfaces where it is brought into contact with Candida, such as in the intestinal tract. It may also be taken in liquid form to attack Candida flourishing in the oesophagus and the mouth. In women, the tendency for Candida to occur in the vagina can be effectively dealt with by the use of vaginal suppositories.

The usual starting dosage of nystatin is one tablet, four times daily, taken in conjunction with the liquid form and suppositories. The dosage is increased to eight tablets daily, after three to six weeks. It can be increased up to a maximum of sixteen tablets daily, after a further three, to six weeks, if required. If no additional benefit is derived at this level the dosage should be reduced to that at which maximum relief from symptoms is achieved.

Initial side effects can sometimes occur when nystatin therapy is commenced. These can be in the form of an exacerbation of symptoms because the body can, initially, be overloaded by the toxic effects of dead Candida cells until they are eliminated. This lasts a few days only and is known as a Herxheimer Reaction. Within two or three weeks a great improvement is felt and chronic symptoms that have existed for years begin to disappear. Food and chemical intolerances become a thing of the past and sense of good health and well-being returns.

Professor Jeffrey Bland from the Department of Biochemistry at the University of Puget Sound, Washington State, has found that there are alternatives to the use of anti-yeast medication. These are:

Lactobacillus Acidophilus — A friendly bacterium used to reinoculate the bowel. Extremely successful in reducing Candida in the intestinal tract. Dosage is one teaspoon three times per day of the dry culture.

Biotin — One of the B vitamins. Three hundred mcgs are taken orally three times per day. Japanese researchers have found that biotin prevents Candida converting to its fungal form.

Oleic Acid — this should be given along with biotin in the form of two teaspoons of olive oil, three times per day.

Copper Aspirinate — The above regimen may have to be continued for a period of up to six months. Once the organism has been converted back to its harmless form, copper aspirinate is taken to facilitate the healing of the gastrointestinal mucosa. This should be taken for about three weeks, to dispel gut inflammation, and then withdrawn. The dosage is one copper aspirinate tablet per day which consists of 10 mg of copper and 330 mg of salicylate.

There is no doubt that candidiasis, in a previously unknown, systemic form, is the cause of suffering for a great number of people with multiple food and chemical allergies. Lack of awareness of this problem by general practitioners is the biggest obstacle to many chronically ill people being diagnosed and effectively treated. Fortunately research is continuing overseas and researchers such as Professor Max Shepherd, of Otago University, are working to develop an effective remedy for this debilitating condition which affects so many people in the community today.

Meanwhile, avoidance of aggravating drugs and foods, together with nystatin, or other anti-fungal therapy, is guaranteed to result in a dramatic improvement in the health of affected individuals. Anyone suffering a range of chronic, undiagnosed symptoms should investigate the possibility of candidiasis-caused multiple allergy illness.

Foods to be eliminated if you are sensitive to moulds or fungi

Mouldy foods consist of spoiled (intentionally or accidentally), fermented, aged or smoked foods.

Cheese of all kinds, including cottage cheese.

Sour cream, sour milk and buttermilk.

Old milk.

Alcoholic liquors, especially beer and wine.

Vinegar and vinegar-containing foods, such as mayonnaise and other salad dressings, chili sauce, pickles, pickled beets, relishes, green olives and sauerkraut.

Pickled and smoked meats and fish, including delicatessen foods, especially frankfurts, corned beef and pickled tongue.

All breads, including pumpernickel, coffee cakes and other foods made with large amounts of yeast, especially Vegemite.

Refined flours and sugars.

Cider and home-made root beer.

Mushrooms.

All dried fruits such as apricots, dates, prunes, figs and raisins.

Canned tomatoes, tomato paste, ketchup, pizza, spaghetti, etc.

Canned juice, especially apple and tomato.

Eat only freshly opened canned foods.

Buy meat fresh daily if possible, or freeze meat as soon as it is brought home. Freezing retards the growth of mould. Avoid foods if made from leftovers such as hash and croquettes. Hamburger moulds very rapidly so use only if made from freshly-ground meat.

6

COELIAC DISORDERS

Being allergic to grains

Allergy illness, in the main, comes about through contact, inhalation or ingestion. Substances harmful to the individual enter the body by these means and overwhelm the immune system causing toxic overload and resulting in various symptoms ranging from mild to severe.

Of the three, ingestion — the eating process — is probably the most suspect due to the great number of different foods and substances contained in the modern diet. Most people have some degree of food intolerance with which their body can cope. Others however, can have severe and constant food allergy problems which keep them chronically ill without apparent cause.

In all cases of food intolerance the small intestine plays a key role by either being unable to function properly, due to damage by the food substance itself; or by other damage due to incorrect feeding in infancy, or by genetic damage due to hereditary factors.

In the case of coeliac disease, a genetic deficiency, in the cellular make-up of the small intestine, can result in partial or total intolerance to gluten. This is a substance found in wheat and rye and, to a lesser extent, in barley and oats. As a result of this intolerance, the mucosa, or mucous membrane, lining the small intestine, loses its villi. These are microscopic, finger-like projections whose job it is to extract nutrients from food and pass them through the intestinal wall into the bloodstream. Once in the bloodstream, the nutrients feed the body and maintain good health. However, if the villi are damaged, the body can no longer receive its proper supply of nutrients, (eg. vitamins, minerals and amino acids). A process of undernourishment is then set in motion, leading to malnutrition and chronic ill health. This process may take many years. During the course of the illness the body becomes increasingly intolerant to a range of foodstuffs, resulting in multiple allergy illness which increases symptoms and worsens the coelic condition.

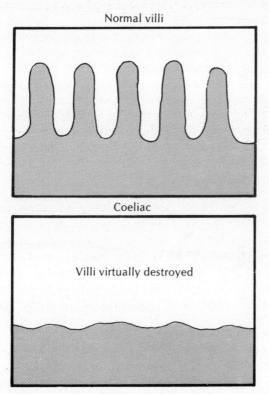

Normal villi

Coeliac

Villi virtually destroyed

Lack of Villi severely reduces the absorption of nutrients — particularly causing deficiencies in Vitamines A, B Group, D, E, K, Protein, Folic Acid, Iron, Calcium and Vitamin B12.

47

Whilst 'coeliac', in its strictest medical sense may refer to gluten intolerance only, in more general terms it means, simply, 'of or in the abdominal cavity'. It is significant, therefore, that the term is given the wider usage in this chapter, because, whereas full-blown gluten intolerance is comparatively rare, there are varying degrees of gluten and/or grain sensitivities, that are comparatively common.

History of coeliac disease

The ancient physician, who recognized and recorded the disease, was known as Aretaeus of Cappadocia and was a contemporary of the great Roman physician of that time, Galen. In 1856, Francis Adams translated Aretaeus' writings for the Sydenham Society of Great Britain. The ancient Greek text used the world *KOILIAKOS*, from which the word coeliac is derived. It means, literally, 'suffering in the bowels'. Aretaeus appears to have understood a great deal about the illness. In his essay on the 'Cure of Coeliacs', he said, 'If the stomach be irretentive of the food and if it passes through undigested and crude, and nothing ascends into the body, we call such persons coeliacs.' He indicated that food made from grains was particularly suspect '... for bread is rarely suitable for giving [coeliac children] strength'.

In 1888, Dr Samuel Gee wrote a paper on the coeliac condition in which he said: 'To regulate the food is the main part of the treatment ... the allowance of farinaceous foods must be *small* ... but if the patient can be cured at all it must be by means of diet.'

A book was written by Dr Herter in 1908 which investigated the problem of coeliac disease in children. Dr Herter said that, in coeliacs, fats were better tolerated than carbohydrates. It was this contention that coeliacs were sensitive to carbohydrates in general, but grains in particular, that was supported by Sir Frederick Still in his memorial lecture to the Royal College of Physicians in 1918, when he said: 'Unfortunately, one form of starch, which seems particularly liable to aggravate the symptoms, is bread. I know of no adequate substitute.'

Dr Howland, in a far-sighted address to the American Paediatric Society, in 1921, on 'Prolonged Intolerance to Carbohydrates' spoke about the health risks of carbohydrates.

From clinical experience it has been found that of all the elements of food, carbohydrate is the one which must be excluded rigorously; that with this greatly reduced, the other elements are almost always well-adjusted even though the absorption of fat may not be so satisfactory as in health.

He advocated a three-stage diet 'with the most careful observation of the digestive capacity ... Bread, cereals and potatoes are the last articles which can be allowed'. He went on to say: 'The treatment is *time-consuming* but these patients will repay the effort expended on them.' I fear that his entreaty to spend more time on *observing* the patient, would fall on very deaf medical ears today.

Dr Haas, in 1938, noted that fatty diarrhoea was experienced by coeliacs with even minute amounts of carbohydrate in the diet and hardly any fatty foods. He found however, that bananas were an excellent form of carbohydrate for coeliacs and caused no diarrhoea or other symptoms.

Since 1950, Professor Dicke, Professor Anderson and others have shown that the exclusion of wheat, rye, oats and barley from the diet of coeliac children, and the substitution of gluten-free products, has reduced inflammation in the small intestine and, in most cases, allowed a return to good health. However, if the gluten-containing cereals were incorporated back into the diet, serious health problems followed in a very short time, due to the lining of the small intestine becoming rapidly abnormal.

Coeliac disease in children

A coeliac disorder can manifest itself at any age. In children it usually becomes evident three to five months after commencing eating gluten-containing foods. In the worst cases, the infant will refuse his feeds, stop putting on weight, become irritable, or listless and develop a large abdomen. Stools become abnormal, either large, pale and offensive or developing into diarrhoea.

In other cases, no symptoms are shown until later in childhood when lack of growth and poor appetite become evident. Tests will indicate excess fat in stools and lack of protein and iron in the blood. A possible diagnosis can be established by passing a tube through the mouth into the upper part of the small intestine and obtaining a tiny piece of its mucosa lining. Examination under a microscope can sometimes show whether degeneration of the villi has taken place.

It has been found in recent years that this procedure does not always show the existence of coeliac disease, leading to conjecture that gluten/wheat intolerance may be far more prevalent than has been traditionally accepted. Therefore, irrespective of the result, a biopsy should be further verified by the use of a low carbohydrate, grain and gluten-free diet, for one or two months. An improvement in health will verify the existence of coeliac disease. Once this disease has been established, the removal of all gluten-containing foods from the diet will ensure a swift recovery. In addition, it may be necessary to restrict fats and sugars for a month or two, until the villi have begun to recover. Full recovery should take place after two to twelve months on a gluten-free diet. Once recovery is advanced, many allergy-type symptoms will disappear as the intestine loses its sensitivity to previously untolerated foods.

It is absolutely essential that a gluten-free diet be maintained permanently. Teenagers, who have been on a gluten-free diet for a number of years, may feel well enough to commence eating normal flour products again. This is a serious mistake and will eventually lead to a breakdown in health caused by renewed damage to the small intestine, and resulting in slowly increasing malabsorption of essential nutrients (vitamins, minerals and amino acids). It may be one or two years before actual symptoms are again experienced, but eventually, unless the gluten-free diet is resumed, chronic illness and stoppage of growth will result.

Coeliac disease in adults

Unfortunately, coeliac disease in adults is neither as easily recognizable nor as quickly recovered from, as in children. Usually it is a less obvious form of the disease which was not apparent during childhood. Even so, the person concerned may have been quite sick since early infancy. Usually such a person either has a history of chronic illnesses which he or she was expected to 'grow out of', or is underdeveloped to some degree, with a tendency towards lethargy and depression.

Because of the time span, coeliac disease, diagnosed in adulthood, will usually have resulted in a greater degree of damage to the small intestine than that occurring in childhood. Some adult coeliacs will only partly respond to a gluten-free diet, due to extensive damage to the small intestine over such a long period. In these cases, almost 5 per cent, corticosteroids have been used with some success. In the great majority of cases however, rigid abstention from grains and gluten, together with reduced intake of refined carbohydrates, revolutionises the sufferer's health and is the only treatment necessary. Supplements of vitamins, minerals and amino acids, taken especially during the first twelve months of a gluten-free diet, will speed up the recovery process.

Unfortunately, the incidence of cancer in patients with adult coeliac disease that remains undetected, is high, up to about 13 per cent. Lymphoma and carcinoma of the small intestine can be fatal complications of this distressing illness. Other illnesses, as potentially serious, can develop as a result of allergy overload due to increasing intolerance by the small intestine to a wide range of foods and substances.

Symptoms

Available evidence suggests that symptoms fall equally into two broad categories. In some cases, they can arise directly from the effects of gluten on the small intestine, such as diarrhoea or abdominal fullness, discomfort, pain and vomiting. The remainder, however, do not experience these specific symptoms to any marked degree. Instead, they complain of a more general malaise involving chronic fatigue, irritability, depression and perhaps, breathlessness. Inevitably, all coeliacs develop intolerances, or allergies, to several foods and chemicals. These allergies will, in turn, cause further symptoms and degeneration of health.

The severity of the illness, and the symptoms experienced, depend on how the small intestine has been affected. As already stated, the abnormality that characterises the coeliac, is damage to the villi in the gut. Usually, this is more evident in the upper part of the small intestine: the part closest to the stomach. The concentration of gluten, being highest here, causes the greatest damage. As it passes down the small intestine, more and more becomes absorbed. Because little or no gluten remains at the lower end, this part of the gut is usually fairly normal. However it is a matter of degree. The greater the damage along the intestine, the more severe will be both symptoms and illness.

The first signs of coeliac disease typically appear in infancy, after weaning and the introduction of cereals. Often the symptoms disappear in later childhood or adolescence, even though the disease continues to affect health and body. Inevitably, symptoms will reassert themselves between the ages of thirty and sixty in the form of adult coeliac disease. If there is any possibility that your child has this problem do not be fooled by a dissappearance of symptoms. Rarely do people grow out of this illness and by the time it again reveals itself in adulthood, much damage to health and life may have occurred.

It is important to remember that the disease may present itself in either childhood or adulthood. If it does not appear until adulthood it simply means that the disease has remained undetected longer and, as a result, has caused more damage. Most coeliac disease begins in early infancy. When symptoms do manifest themselves in childhood, the following are typical:

The child does not develop as quickly as his siblings and fails to thrive.

Pale, malodorous and bulky stools are often passed.

Abdominal bloating, which may or may not be painful, is often experienced.

The child is pale, querulous and lacks stamina.

The child is plagued by respiratory ailments and other chronic symptoms.

Allergies to some foods, especially milk products, become apparent.

Diarrhoea — occurring often.

In adulthood, further symptoms would be:

Anaemia — particularly during pregnancy.

Bone pain — particularly in the lower legs.

Skin disorders such as dermatitis, herpetiformis (a skin disorder characterised by vesicles and papules which affects the feet and other parts of the body).

Allergies to a number of foods and chemicals.

Chronic tiredness and irritability.

Poor health, in general, and lack of vitality.

Rapid deterioration of health after early middle age.

Treatment

The primary, and most important, treatment is the elimination of grains containing gluten from the diet. In addition, it may be necessary to severely restrict intake of non-glutinous grains and refined carbohydrate. If these rules are not adhered to, a severe relapse, especially in later life, will generally follow. It is therefore essential to avoid eating any food containing wheat, rye, barley and oats. This covers a fairly wide range of foodstuffs, and it is important to read the labels on canned, bottled and packaged foods to ensure that fillers containing gluten, have not been used. For the coeliac, even small amounts of gluten, in the form of breadcrumbs, batter, gravy, sauces, etc., can cause serious damage to the small intestine.

Because of malabsorption of nutrients, due to intestinal damage, a course of supplements is extremely useful in aiding the body to recover. Many coeliacs are found to be anaemic due to deficiencies or iron and folic acid. Calcium deficiency is common and is due partly, to vitamin D deficiency and partly to calcium binding to unabsorbed fatty acids. In general, malabsorption due to coeliac disease, starves the body of most vital nutrients to some degree. Accordingly, it is important to take daily doses of vitamin, mineral and amino acid complexes during the recovery period. If the small intestine of the coeliac has been severely affected, it may always remain delicate. It may well be necessary to continue with some form of nutrient supplementation after recovery, to ensure maintenance of good health.

Some coeliacs may suffer from a lactase deficiency due either to intestinal damage caused by the disease, or reasons such as incorrect feeding during infancy or hereditary factors. It is important that these people exclude milk and milk products from their diet as well as cereals containing gluten. If this problem is not recognized, then a gluten-free diet alone, will not allow a full recovery.

Some sufferers may also have to abstain from refined carbohydrates, such as cereals and sugar, due to the extent of intestinal damage. For these people, essential carbohydrate may be easily obtained from fruit and vegetables, especially bananas. An ongoing diet, along these lines, will save the intestine from further deterioration and ensure a continuing level of health.

Coeliac disease is difficult to diagnose and there is considerable evidence that, due to the overconsumption of grains in our society, it is far more prevalent than previously indicated. It is a prime source of multiple allergy illness and toxic overload due to the damage done to the small intestine, where the bulk of food digestion and assimilation takes place. As well as damage to the villi, the intestinal walls can become porous and allow toxic, partly digested food particles into the bloodstream where they will cause allergy symptoms and wreak havoc on the body's immune system.

It has long been suspected that there are many degrees of coeliac disease, not all of which can be diagnosed effectively by use of the biopsy procedure.

ALLERGY EFFECTS ON THE BODY

Further illness awaits

To counteract the continual toxic assault, to which people unwittingly subject themselves, the vital organs work constantly to detoxify the blood and to eliminate harmful substances from the body. For years, most of these substances are expelled, but those excesses, with which the excretory organs cannot cope, accumulate in all tissues and organs, gradually aging them and depleting their function.

Eventually the liver is incapable of coping fully with its detoxifying duties, with the result that the toxins circulate in the blood to poison the system and damage the kidneys.

From *The New Health Revolution* by Ross Horne.

In previous chapters, reference has been made to the damage caused by accumulated toxins as a result of allergy conditions, particularly masked allergies, remaining undetected for many years. In order to better understand how the body works and which organs are involved in, or affected by, the allergy process, a brief look at some of the appropriate parts of the body is necessary.

Digestive System Organs

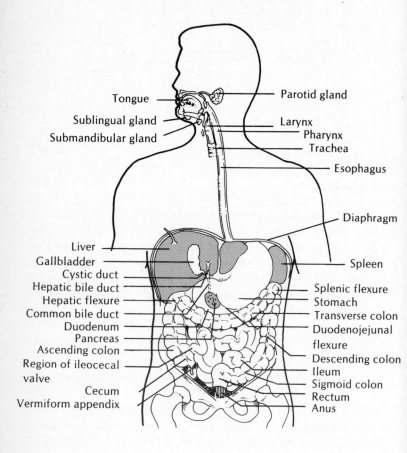

The pancreas

The pancreas is a long, narrow gland which stretches from the spleen to about the middle of the duodenum. It has three main functions. Firstly, to provide digestive juices for everything that goes through the duodenum. These digestive juices contain pancreatic enzymes in an alkaline solution to provide the right conditions for the digestive process to be completed in the small intestine. Secondly, the pancreas produces insulin, the hormone which controls blood sugar by the metabolism of sugar and other carbohydrates. Thirdly, it produces sodium bicarbonate to neutralise acids coming from the stomach and so provide the right environment for the pancreatic enzymes to be effective.

Many people with food and chemical allergy problems have an inability, either to produce a certain enzyme, or to produce enough enzymes for the digestive process to work effectively. In conjunction with this is an inability to produce enough sodium bicarbonate — essential for the pancreatic enzymes to function properly. As a result, partially digested peptides (protein particles) are absorbed into the bloodstream and attach themselves to other proteins, thereby inducing further allergic reactions. The inflammation in the system, resulting from continuing allergic reactions, can focus on a 'target' organ, causing injury and, finally, serious disease. This can often happen to the pancreas, thus the initial malfunction may, not only accentuate an allergic response, but may also lead to further inflammation of the pancreas itself.

Clinical ecologists have discovered that production of insulin by the pancreas is directly related, not only to the intake of carbohydrates, but also to the ingestion of all types of food. They have also noticed that insulin production is altered by allergenic foods. Accordingly, this abnormal insulin reaction can be used to identify the offending allergen, by giving a person a standard dose of the suspected food, or chemical, and observing his blood sugar level after a measured time.

The pancreas therefore is an important organ in the mediation of both addiction and allergy. Very often it is the first organ in the body to be significantly affected by any allergen.

The small intestine

The small intestine is a narrow tube, about six metres long, which empties into the large intestine or colon. It is a vital organ of the body as it carries out most of the digestive processes.

After being mixed with hydrochloric acid in the stomach, food passes through the duodenum into the small intestine. Here, enzymes secreted by the intestinal wall set about the biochemical process of breaking down the food into its various chemical components. Absorption of these components then takes place through the villi, which are tiny finger-like projections in the intestinal wall. In this way the body receives its essential nutrients of vitamins, minerals, amino acids and enzymes.

Food allergy problems usually cause some damage to the small intestine. In the case of grain allergies, this can be serious and even result in death, through intestinal cancer. At best, damage to the villi and intestinal wall will cause malabsorption: a reduction in absorption of essential nutrients. This leads to exacerbation of the allergy problem with further food intolerance developing. The intestinal wall becomes porous and allows undigested food particles to enter the blood stream, causing further havoc to a floundering immune system. Eventually, a complete breakdown in health can occur.

The liver

The liver is the largest gland in the body. Amongst other things, it is a detoxifying agent and a blood reservoir. It breaks down waste matter in the blood and manufactures blood proteins; converting sugar and carbohydrates into glycogen, which it then stores for the manufacture of glucose when needed. It collects vitamins and minerals from food and stores them for future use. The liver also manufactures bile, which is stored in the gall bladder, and released, when necessary, into the duodenum to aid in the digestion of fats.

During digestion, bile flows from the gall bladder and liver into the small intestine, thus helping to keep it alkaline and aiding the pancreatic enzymes to digest fats more easily. Eventually the bile fluids circulate back to the liver, from the colon, carrying toxins with them. These must be neutralised by the liver and, finally, eliminated by the kidneys.

The allergic reaction creates turmoil in the body when antibodies and antigens react, causing mast cells to break up and histamine to be released in large quantities. These adverse chemical reactions result in the body becoming overloaded with toxins which eventually find their way to the colon for elimination. Unfortunately, the constipation, which is so often present in allergy conditions, causes these toxins to remain in the colon. This results in the bile fluids continuously overloading the liver with recirculated toxins from the colon and eventually, the liver may become incapable of coping fully with its detoxifying duties. When this happens, the liver degenerates, the system becomes poisoned and the individual, who has never been well because of masked allergies, now becomes seriously ill.

The effects, therefore, of allergies, particularly several masked allergies, on the liver, over a period of time, can be extremely serious and cause further severe illness.

The colon

The colon is the main part of the large intestine and consists of the ascending colon, the transverse colon, the descending colon and the sigmoid colon. It is a muscular tube which carries food residue (chyme) from the cecum (the first part of the large intestine) to the rectum (the last part). The first half of the colon, from the cecum to the middle of the transverse colon, is responsible for the creation of wavelike motions known as peristaltic waves, which push the contents of the colon to the rectum for eventual evacuation.

Besides the formation of peristaltic waves, the first half of the colon also extracts from the chyme, any available nutritional material, including water, that the small intestine was unable to collect. For this purpose, it mulches the chyme and transfers liquid and nutrients through its walls into the bloodstream. This is done through the blood vessels lining the walls of the colon, which then transfer the nutrients back to the liver for processing.

Constipation, which often accompanies food allergies, causes the accumulation of fecal matter in the colon which proceeds to putrify and ferment. Combine this with the additional wastes caused by the body's continuing allergic responses, and an overloaded toxic situation occurs in the colon, with devastating effects. The colon is faced with the extraction of remaining nutrients from fermenting, toxin-laden rubbish. As a result, polluted nutrients pass back into the bloodstream to aggravate further the allergy condition.

Urinary System Organs

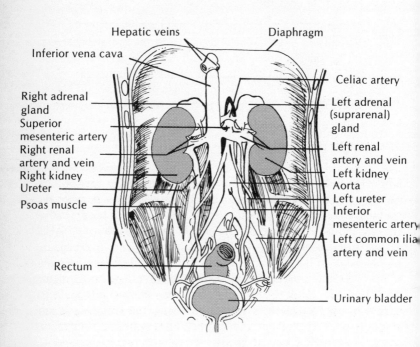

Hepatic veins

Diaphragm

Inferior vena cava

Celiac artery

Right adrenal gland

Left adrenal (suprarenal) gland

Superior mesenteric artery

Right renal artery and vein

Left renal artery and vein

Right kidney

Left kidney

Ureter

Aorta

Psoas muscle

Left ureter

Inferior mesenteric artery

Left common iliac artery and vein

Rectum

Urinary bladder

The kidneys

The two kidneys are responsible for many vital functions. Briefly, they perform the complex task of extracting from the blood, used up proteins, minerals and other elements making up the toxic waste of the metabolic process. This residual material, together with waste water, is then passed in the form of urine, through to the bladder before being finally expelled from the body.

Allergy-caused overloading may cause the liver to deteriorate and lose its capacity to cope fully with its detoxifying duties. As a result, the toxins, left to circulate in the blood, will poison the body and cause damage to the kidneys. Recent studies have shown that kidney failure can be caused by overloading with food toxins. Since undetected food allergies are known to overload the body with toxins, it follows that the kidneys will indeed suffer and may become a 'target' organ.

The respiratory system

The respiratory system comprises the trachea (windpipe), the bronchials and the lungs. Air that we breathe passes through the trachea and bronchials into the lungs where it is used to oxygenate the blood. At the same time, carbon dioxide is extracted from the blood and expelled from the lungs into the atmosphere.

Victims of ecological allergies invariably suffer from chemical as well as food intolerances. Some of the more common chemical allergens are the hydrocarbon products, such as petrol and diesel fumes, pressure pack propellants, etc. When these substances are inhaled into the lungs they are absorbed along with oxygen into the bloodstream. To the allergic person, this ingestion through the lungs sets up the same allergic process as an allergy reaction, caused by eating an allergenic food. Consequently, the person becomes ill but often does not realize the cause, since chemical allergies, like food allergies, can be masked, with resultant symptoms that are seemingly unrelated to the chemicals concerned.

An example of food allergies causing respiratory symptoms is found in a report from Dr Elmer Cranton, of Virginia, who says that recurrent coughs are due to food allergies, not colds. This view

Respiratory System Organs

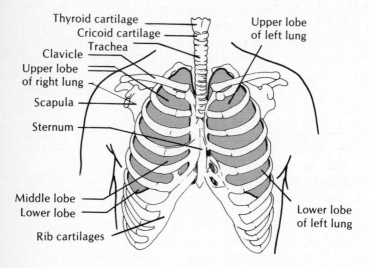

was also recently supported by the *British Medical Journal*. Dr Cranton said that the most likely causes were dairy products, yeast, wheat products, eggs and citrus fruit. He has found with people allergic to these foods, that once they have been removed from the diet, the coughing stops.

Milk and milk products are one of the commonest causes of food allergies. Often, the reaction is a general tendency for excessive mucus to form in the nasal and other respiratory passages. This, in

62

turn, can lead to constant colds, sore throats, nasal catarrh and asthma — all by-products of an ongoing and debilitating food allergy.

The stomach

The stomach is a simple, bag-like organ and is part of the alimentary canal. It lies between the esophagus and the small intestine. The upper end of the stomach connects with the esophagus, whilst the lower end opens into the doudenum, which is the upper part of the small intestine. The stomach serves as a storage place for food, enabling a large meal to be eaten at one time. It also produces hydrochloric acid and the enzyme pepsin, to digest the food partially.

There are a number of different foods that will irritate the mucous membrane lining the stomach. Highly spiced foods, extremely hot foods and alcoholic drinks can cause ulcers to develop in the stomach or duodenum. Another cause of stomach ulcers can be the regular ingestion of foods to which the person is allergic. It is interesting to note, that the Japanese have the highest rate of stomach cancer in the world, due to the high salt content in their diet.

Dr James Brennan, in his book, *Basics of Food Allergy,* says that some ulcers are actually a symptom of milk allergy. He discovered this after treating a patient of his who had a duodenal ulcer for over ten years. He found that, by putting his patient on a diet which excluded many of the allergenic foods, the ulcer symptoms disappeared within three days. One by one, various foods were then added back into the diet to see which food caused the allergy. When milk was added to the diet the patient suffered abdominal pain, vomiting and weakness. Once it was again removed from the diet the symptoms disappeared.

Dr Brennan went on to discover, by the same process, that his patient's ulcer was also inflamed by wheat and pork. Once these foods were permanently removed, the patient remained symptom-free for sixteen years.

Other doctors have found that, after removing chocolate, coffee and other known allergenic foods from their patients diets, stomach ulcers have disappeared. Dr Albert Rowe, co-author of *Food Allergy,* has found that eliminating eggs from a person's diet can greatly assist ulcer conditions.

There seems no doubt that stomach and duodenal ulcers are yet another symptom of the chronic masked food allergy.

Hypoglycaemia

Hypoglycaemia is commonly found in people suffering from masked food allergies. It occurs when the body does not have enough blood sugar.

If a person has eaten excessive carbohydrate, over many years, especially refined carbohydrate such as white flour and sugar, the pancreas becomes stressed to the point where it ceases to operate normally — a very common problem today. These eating habits alter the normal, gentle production of insulin by the pancreas to that of rapid insulin output because of the excessive demands placed on it by so much carbohydrate. The human body was simply not designed to deal with the excessive amounts of carbohydrate in our so-called civilized diet. The pancreas becomes used to producing excessive amounts of insulin to cope with the large rises in blood sugar, brought about by constant carbohydrate ingestion. Finally, it becomes overstressed and tired. In this confused state, a small rise in blood sugar will often cause it to produce a disproportionate amount of insulin, resulting in low blood sugar and subsequent hypoglycaemia.

This is of particular importance to sufferers of masked food allergies, which, invariably, involve many of the carbohydrate foods, often in the form of refined carbohydrates, such as cereal flours and refined sugars. The need for these people to snack constantly or 'binge' on their favourite (addictive) foods, coupled with the probability that they have been excessive eaters of these foods for many years, makes them inevitable targets for hypoglycaemia. During the phase of hypoglycaemia, the individual suffers from faintness, palpitations, nausea and excessive sweating. In order to overcome these distressing symptoms, he immediately eats more refined carbohydrate, which in turn stimulates further insulin production, so that the symptoms then return. Thus, a vicious circle becomes established, due to the demands made on the pancreas by the persistent ingestion of refined carbohydrates. This would have been brought about by chronic, addictive, masked allergy to one, or more, foods, which is unknown to the sufferer.

Clinical ecologists can often relate the hypoglycaemic reaction to a specific carbohydrate, by the use of a glucose tolerance test. This allows them to identify the offending allergen, which for years may have been causing untold distress and suffering to the person concerned.

American allergists believe that a drop in blood sugar can be caused by eating foods to which you are, unknowingly, allergic. The reason being that internal stress is caused by any allergic substance. Hormonal stress can cause a fall in blood sugar. Studies in America have discovered that up to 90 per cent of American prison inmates have hypoglycaemia, resulting from poor nutrition. This leads to severe psychological and behavioural problems. Once diets are corrected, a dramatic improvement in attitude can result. These people can be said to be the really unlucky victims of food intolerance. Unfortunately, whilst some prisons are taking steps to improve diet, others are not. Such a case is the Alabama prison which feeds inmates on hamburgers and other fast foods.

Arthritis

Many doctors have refused to accept that both arthritis and rheumatism, are either caused, or at the very least seriously affected, by diet. Most people over the age of thirty, will notice a twinge or an ache somewhere, if they persist in eating something that is bad for them. In actual fact, both rheumatism and arthritis are classic examples of masked food allergies at their rampaging worst. There is a mass of evidence throughout the world to support this fact.

One example, in many, is research done during a three and a half year clinical trial, conducted by Dr D.M. Carroll of North Carolina. In 300 patients suffering from rheumatoid arthritis, 98 per cent were found to be severly allergic to different foods, and some to several foods. The analysis showed 37 per cent allergic to wheat, 27 per cent to corn, 23 per cent to milk, 19 per cent to eggs and 12 per cent to tomatoes. Once the offending foods were removed from their diets, they all showed marked improvement. That is very conclusive evidence in one study.

The influence of arthritis on our society is significant. In 1981, according to the Bureau of Statistics, it was responsible for 25 per cent more lost work time than industrial disputes. It is known to affect 1,250,000 Australians, many of them children. Common sense must eventually dictate that the diet and environment of these people, should be thoroughly examined for food and chemical intolerances.

At present the most widespread medical treatment for arthritis is the administration of large daily doses of aspirin, over a prolonged period. Aspirin is made up of acetylsalicylic acid which is a salicylate derivative. It is well documented that salicylates are a potent allergen, affecting many people. Could this not then be a case of masking the disease with the very substance which is causing it?

This chapter is not meant to be an exhaustive examination of all allergy effects on the human body. There is virtually no part of the body which may not be affected, either directly or indirectly, by an allergic reaction — particularly with respect to food and chemical intolerances. It is important to understand that the effects of an ongoing allergic condition, on the body, can ultimately be catastrophic, by virtue of the cumulative effects over months or years. These effects certainly go much further than the general, discomforting symptoms discussed in previous chapters and can lead to serious degeneration and disease in major organs if allowed to persist undetected.

Unfortunately, few doctors understand that allergy illness affects the body as a whole. This problem is well described in a passage from the *Complete Book of Homeopathy* by Michael Weiner and Kathleen Goss.

Yet perhaps the most destructive effect of modern orthodox medicine lies in the changes that have taken place between physician and patient ... The general practitioner (in the traditional sense) is almost a thing of the past, and each specialist treats only that organ system that comes within his area of expertise. No wonder we feel that our doctors are not really looking at us as whole beings. Common sense tells us that many symptoms appearing in different organs systems may be related — that they at least constitute a whole picture of our state of health. Yet our trips to the doctor's office must often result in a sense of frustration when we feel that the specific organ-directed treatment we receive is not based upon the doctor's assessment of our entire symptom picture.

8

FOOD ALLERGIES

A major source of ill-health

People are getting sick, in fact chronically ill, simply by eating the foods that they have been brought up to believe are good for them. As doctors continue to experience growing numbers of patients with a wide range of recurring symptoms, the medical fraternity will have to acknowledge the affect of diet on their patients' health.

In England, recently, Professor Maurice Lessoff completed an inquiry into food allergies for the Royal College of Physicians. He said that such illnesses are common and should be taken seriously. He found that, often, people with genuine food allergies are wrongly told they have a psychological problem. How many people have been forced to lead miserable lives because narrow-minded doctors are unwilling to accept food allergy as a major cause of illness! This situation is extraordinary when you consider that 2400 years ago Hippocrates, the great Greek physician, said that the most important thing, of which a doctor should take note, is his patient's food and drink and the effects of these things on his health.

The almost universal consumption of highly refined foods, in the West, has become a serious problem. Take-away foods eaten daily by many people are particularly dangerous as they have been processed, flavoured and tenderised with a sickening array of artificial substances. The problem is one of degree. The human body can withstand the onslaught of a considerable amount of the processed toxic rubbish, contained in the Western diet. However, there comes a time when it cannot continue to do so. It simply becomes overloaded and begins to break down. This may happen at any time in life — from childhood onwards and to any person who persists in eating the modern, universally processed Western foods. High fibre additives are not enough. These do not act as an antidote for all the manufactured foods and substances that are, literally, wearing out the body.

Food allergies in childhood

A major study conducted in the United Kingdom and reported in the *Archives of Disease in Childhood*, examined children suffering from vomiting, diarrhoea, colic, abdominal pain, eczema and urticaria (hives). It found that 40 per cent were sensitive to cow's milk, with the remainder being affected by a wide range of other intolerances.

Dr W. Allan Walker of Massachusetts General Hospital, has found that chemical substances from the mother, passed to the infant in breast milk, will prevent foreign substances from passing through the baby's underdeveloped intestinal wall. Babies are extremely vulnerable during the first few weeks after birth and are unable to make the protective substances that guard their intestinal and respiratory tracts from foreign invaders. Particularly during the first few days of life, it is essential that a baby receive colostrum from its mother, which coats the intestinal wall and acts as an undercoat protection. Without colostrum, and other antibodies in the mother's milk, infants will invariably be badly affected by foreign particles entering the bloodstream, to wreak immunological havoc in their tiny bodies. The resultant damage is very often permanent. Cow's milk is the most common foreign protein to cause damage and, in recent years, it has been realized that many people, who are now adults, have been damaged during their infant feeding. The result is often a lifetime sensitivity to cow's milk and other foods and chemicals.

Dr Paul Buisseret, of Guy's Hospital Medical School, London, in a study of seventy-nine allergic children, found severe behavioural problems in at least a third of the children studied. Once cow's milk was withdrawn, these problems gradually subsided over a period of some weeks. Even babies being fed on breast milk are not always free of cow's milk allergy. Dr Irene Jakobsen and Dr Tor Lindberg, of the University of Lund, Sweden, described eighteen mothers of infants who suffered from colic. The colic disappeared when the mothers were put on diets free of cow's milk. Evidently, proteins in the cow's milk were getting to the baby through the mother's breast.

Food allergies can commence during the first six months of life. If children are introduced too early to cow's milk, cereals, orange juice and other substances, such as those contained in manufactured baby food, there is a great danger that they may become intolerant to those foods, and will remain so, for the rest of their lives. This paints a bleak scenario for the child. It will mean that throughout childhood, he will be encouraged by well-meaning parents to eat foods which are semi-poisonous to him. As a result, the child will develop chronic medical symptoms. In some fortunate cases, the symptom or symptoms may be easily linked to a specific food. For example, the child may react quickly, after eating an orange or drinking a glass of milk, with a hay fever attack or vomiting. More often than not, however, the child will exhibit a continuous range of symptoms such as irritability, lethargy, respiratory infections and catarrh, to name but a few.

The well-meaning parents then proceed to consult doctors and specialists throughout the early life of the child. In time, they may be advised to remove a food from the child's diet to see if there is an improvement. Sometimes there is and the problem is solved — luckily for the child. However, often it is not so simple. The child, having been exposed to several foreign substances too early in his development, may have developed more than one allergy. The removal of one food may not cause the symptoms to go away, as this allergy is masked by the others. This results in the child being allowed to recommence eating a food, which, amongst others, is making him ill. Eventually, the child is classified, by doctors and parents alike, as 'prone' or 'delicate' and his activities are restricted accordingly.

The problem is further complicated by the child appearing to 'grow out' of the symptoms at some future stage in his development. There could be several reasons for this. Firstly, as the child gets older and stronger his system becomes more robust and, for a while, may overcome the allergenic poisoning being done to him. However, it may be just a matter of time before other illness or injury may overstress the immune system, causing it to break down again. Secondly, he may, through a change of diet and habits simply stop eating the offending food. This can happen when the child has become old enough to assert himself. If addiction to the allergen has not set in, he may be in a position to reject instinctively the food as being bad for him. This rejection would be strengthened in his subconscious by the resultant immediate improvement in health.

Parents should take note of a child's constant rejection of a known allergy-causing food. This is often the first sign that the child has some sensitivity to it. The child, after being forced to eat the food for a while, will most likely overcome his instinctive aversion and, instead, develop an addiction to it. Whilst the parents may think that their child is finally co-operating, he has in actual fact, become 'hooked' and a masked addiction/allergy process, with a range of perplexing symptoms, has begun.

Food allergies in adulthood

In Chapter 2, the process of ecological illness, leading to multiple allergies, was discussed. It has become evident that many people in the Western World are developing chronic illness as a result of too many years on the over-refined Western diet. It appears that, although people who were fed wrongly during infancy are particularly prone to developing this problem, most people, in fact, will develop some form of ecologically-caused food intolerances during the course of their lives. The fact that this problem has not emerged *en masse* sooner, in our society, is probably because it is only during the past thirty years that manufactured and artificially processed foods have become the bulk of our daily diet.

The process of ecological illness can span years, even decades. That incredible mechanism, the body, can put up a very good fight for a very long time. The individual, being a fighter, keeps plugging along, coping with repetitive ailments, little realizing that he is inexorably developing a condition that will ultimately wreck his health. These days, once a person moves past thirty-five, it seems that a range of repetitive ailments, from backache to indigestion, have to be accepted as part of the ageing process. The fact that the body is becoming increasingly overloaded and is giving out warning signs, does not often appear to be recognized nor understood. These warnings are often the first signs of a weakening immune system, which if unheeded, will lead to complex food and chemical allergies, causing a further breakdown in health.

Dr Allen G. Grant of Charing Cross Hospital, London, reported, in the *Lancet*, on the study of sixty migraine patients. It was found that 78 per cent were allergic to wheat, 65 per cent to oranges, 40 per cent to tea and coffee, 45 per cent to eggs, 37 per cent to chocolate and milk, 35 per cent to beef, and 33 per cent to corn, cane sugar and yeast. Dr Grant found that, if these foods were eliminated from their diet, 85 per cent became free of headaches and the rest showed significant improvement. This work was supported by research at the National Hospital for Nervous Diseases, in London, where it was found that at least two thirds of severe migraine sufferers were allergic to certain foods. When these foods were removed from the diet, the headaches stopped.

Many elderly people, nowadays, are showing signs of ecological illness because their immune systems are less robust than a younger person's and the effects of the past thirty years have hit them first. They are told by their doctors that they must accept their recurring symptoms and their chronic fatigue, simply because they are getting old. They are not advised to examine their diet or eating habits and, accordingly, their later years are unnecessarily burdened with ill health. It has been shown overseas that a clean diet, free from processed and allergenic foods, can rebuild the immune system and, within a dramatically short time, restore elderly people to robust good health. Nathan Pritikin's now famous Longevity Centre, at Santa Monica, California, has been enormously successful in this field.

As time goes on, many younger people are beginning to show signs of the ecological allergy syndrome. Doctors' waiting rooms are evidencing increasing numbers of young people in their twenties and even younger, with recurring symptoms and health problems. Why is the percentage of young patients higher than, say twenty years ago? It seems that a growing intolerance to our artificial Western diet is the answer.

Allergenic foods

Overloading the body with too many processed foods, with their chemical additives, for too long, can cause an eventual breakdown in health in even the most robust person. The individual, besides developing a 'general intolerance' to processed foods, will often become extremely allergic to one or a number of the well-known allergenic foods. The tragedy is that these allergies can be masked, or hidden, within the range of symptoms which begin to exhibit themselves due to a developing 'general intolerance'.

A reaction to a specific food can either be immediate, or delayed, depending on the degree of sensitisation to the allergen and whether it has reached the gut, in the form of digested or undigested material. This is dependent on whether the immune system is functioning correctly and/or the appropriate enzyme is being manufactured by the body. For example, an allergen in digested material, such as cereals, can make itself felt up to twenty-four hours after the meal, whereas an undigested material, such as egg white, may have an immediate reaction. Even then, depending on the severity and duration of the reaction, unless the egg white is eaten by itself, other foods may confuse the issue, especially if there are other allergenic foods amongst them.

Foods known to be common causes of allergies are:-

Milk and dairy products
Cereal and grain products (especially wheat)
Eggs
Fish
Sugar
Yeast
Citrus fruits
Tomatoes
Mushrooms
Pork (including ham and bacon)
Chocolate, cocoa etc.
Coffee and tea

Nuts
Packaged food
Tinned food
Frozen food
All alcohol (especially red wine and beer)

Although these are the more widely recognized allergenic foods, once the immune system becomes overloaded, virtually any food can become an allergy problem.

A recent survey in the United States came up with some startling facts. It concluded that forty million Americans constantly suffer from the more commonly recognized allergy symptoms of hay fever, asthma and skin disease. It also suggested that the old chestnuts of dust, cats, pollen etc. being responsible, were in fact only minor causes compared with the large numbers of people affected by food allergies.

Two major foods, which constantly cause allergic reactions today, are dairy products and grain products. These have been staple foods of the human race for thousands of years. Why, then, should milk and cereals, and their derivatives, become the cause of so much illness in the latter part of the twentieth century? If you stop and think about it, the answer is obvious. These foods are not the foods that our forebears ate.

Milk

Dr Maurice Bowerman, of Oregon, in a paper written in 1980, described the damaging effect of milk on five of his patients, who for years had suffered from fatigue, poor memory and poor concentration. When milk was removed from their diets, four patients became free of symptoms and the fifth greatly improved. Why is milk so damaging? One reason is 'pasteurization'.

When milk is pasteurized, the natural enzymes present in raw milk are destroyed. Without these enzymes, milk cannot be properly digested. One of the most important enzymes in milk is lipase, which is there to break down fat. Pasteurized milk no longer has this enzyme and this makes it impossible for the body to digest it properly. As a result, undigested milk particles can end up in the bloodstream causing havoc to the immune system and resulting in a confusing array of allergy reactions. Apart from the fact that cow's milk is four times stronger than breast milk, infants fed on cow's milk, also have to contend with the enormous task of digesting it. No wonder many of them get sick, and remain sick, throughout their lives until milk is removed from their diet.

Pasteurized cow's milk is particularly damaging to infants under twelve months of age. It has been found to cause gastrointestinal blood loss due to the effect on the baby's underdeveloped intestinal tract. Cow's milk is also too high in protein, sodium, and potassium for a baby's immature kidneys and, thus places them under great strain. Anaemia may develop because of the child's low iron content, combined with blood loss from the intestine. These problems can continue in later life.

Professor Carl Wood, an eminent medical academic and chairman of the in vitro fertilization programme, at the Queen Victoria Medical Centre in Melbourne found that his allergy to milk was leading to a variety of symptoms.

I used to get gastro-enterological problems — a lot of diarrhoea, colic, also fuzziness and tiredness after a meal, and all that was related to the fact that I can't tolerate milk. After some years of taking milk when you can't tolerate it you become very sensitive to all sorts of foods. So I have a very basic diet — steamed vegies and simple meats and I feel much better.

A classic example of how a milk allergy can hoodwink a doctor, even one of Professor Wood's stature — and cause further food allergies to develop.

It must be understood that milk includes all dairy products and foods, containing milk as an additive. An allergy to milk usually requires total abstinence from foods containing it, in order to stay well.

Cereals and grains

Forty years ago, Dr Edward Howell, of Chicago, described extensive research into the eating habits of Malays and Filipinos. He found that these people, who subsisted mainly on rice, had all developed hypertrophy of the pancreas.

Further studies since then have shown that large consumption of other grain products has the same effect. Hypertrophy of the pancreas is enlargement, due to overwork, over a long period of time. Grain products are impossible to digest raw and must be cooked, or processed, first. Even then, large amounts of pancreatic enzymes are needed to consume them which can often lead to a tired and inefficient pancreas from middle life onwards. The message is clear; do not eat grain and cereal products every day. They should be eaten sparingly, to provide diversity, not bulk.

Allergy sufferers will often find they are allergic to wheat and, perhaps, other grains, such as oats and corn. If they have been big eaters of these foods in the past, their overworked pancreas may no longer be coping efficiently. As a result undigested particles are reaching their bloodstream and causing allergic reactions, often in the form of masked, recurring symptoms which appear to have no relativity to bread or other grain food concerned. Sensitivity to grains can be further aggravated by the bleaching agents used in white flour and other chemicals used in the modern refining and milling process.

Dr Abraham Hoffer, a renowned Canadian psychiatrist and nutritionist, commented, at a recent Australian seminar, on the effects of reduced cereal intake in European countries during both World Wars. He pointed out that, before the invention of agriculture, humans had been hunter/gatherers, but now consumed too many cereal products, especially refined breads and flours. During both wars, European countries had problems getting enough wheat from North America and elsewhere. As a result, these countries, including the UK, showed improved health and a much lower rate of admissions to mental hospitals. He said the reason for this was that many people have only a limited capacity for digesting grain products, especially wheat. Therefore, excessive grain consumption for these people (which could simply mean eating bread every day) would result in severe allergy, with such distressing symptoms as schizophrenia, coeliac disease and various gastrointestinal illnesses, including chronic constipation.

In his research Dr Hoffer had found that severe digenerative disease, brought about by intolerance to the excess use of grains in the Western diet, had developed amongst, comparatively healthy, primitive tribes, within a mere twenty years. This was particularly evident in studies of the Kung, in Southern Africa, the Australian Aborigines and the Prima Indians of Arizona.

The cereal problem, has been further aggravated by the fact that, since the Second World War, babies have invariably been weaned onto cereals far too early in their development. For many people, this has resulted in permanent damage to the intestinal lining, with subsequent impairment of digestion. As a result, not only do they have a lifelong allergy to cereals, but they can suffer from poor absorption of nutrients generally and require daily supplements to keep in reasonable health. Abstinence from cereals is vital for these people, if they wish to remain well.

CHEMICAL ALLERGIES

Our greatest danger?

In previous chapters, brief reference has been made to the encroachment of chemicals into our everyday lives. Never in the history of mankind has there been a period to compare with the chemical barrage of the past thirty years.

Civilization has entered a new era, an era of convenience and expediency, in which virtually every aspect of our lives contains a seemingly unavoidable association with chemicals of one kind or another. For years, we have been subjected to every conceivable form of marketing and advertising, designed to convince us that the incredible array of manufactured, processed, tinned, packaged and bottled foods are superior to the fresh, natural foods of our forefathers. The processing removes most of the natural goodness and flavour of the food and it is turned into an almost indigestible form due to the complete absence of natural enzymes — destroyed through processing and cooking. Regular ingestion of these foods over a period of years, places an extreme load on the pancreas, liver and digestive system, as a whole, causing the body to wear out much sooner than it should.

As if this is not bad enough, further strain is placed on the body by the assortment of chemicals needed to preserve colour, dry,

78

flavour and tenderise processed food, in order to get people to eat it. By this stage, it is not really food but more a composition of reconstituted, chemical-laden organic matter. A recent study has shown that the average person now consumes about three kilograms of chemicals per year, in the form of food additives. The human body was never designed to be so constantly abused. It becomes overloaded and develops allergies to all the unnatural rubbish with which it has been constantly fed. It is again a matter of degree. A little processed food, now and again, is no problem for a healthy body. But, when it is eaten on a daily basis, year after year, as the main ingredients of the diet, the body will lose its capacity to cope, and an insidious form of ill health will result.

An additional source of chemicals, which is still not generally appreciated by the medical profession and others, is the widespread use of pesticides and insecticides. These not only add toxic residues to fruits, vegetables and other food crops, but also contaminate meat and milk. Thus, another burden of toxicity is added to our already overloaded systems, resulting in allergic responses and a hastening of the degenerative disease process.

With pesticides in common use such as DDT, Paraquat and 245T, what chance has the human body, when even fresh food is loaded with chemicals before reaching the table! Awareness of the problem, and avoidance of chemicals wherever possible, is the only answer.

Monosodium Glutamate

One of the principal offenders amongst food additives, is monosodium glutamate, commonly known as MSG. Researchers at Monash University have called for manufacturers to stop adding MSG to food. The use of this toxic chemical to artificially enhance the flavour of tinned food, is so widespread that it is difficult to find any type of canned or processed food that does not contain it. It is commonly used in fast food outlets, the restaurant trade and is particularly favoured by Chinese restaurants. Also it is used in the manufacture of hamburgers, pizzas and sausages. People who experience a reaction to MSG can suffer such symptoms as tightening of the facial muscles, visual disturbances, headache, gastrointestinal pain, fainting, irritability, tiredness, dry mouth and disturbed sleep. These symptoms can be either immediate or delayed. It is now known that MSG slows learning ability, especially when given during the first few weeks of life. (Many tinned baby foods, in the past, have contained MSG). High doses can cause visible brain lesions, whilst low doses upset brain chemistry by triggering nerves which are not meant to be triggered.

Since the early 1970's it has been known that MSG causes health problems and yet this particularly nasty, highly toxic chemical is still to be found in a huge variety of processed foods commonly eaten by people every day of their lives. This is an extraordinary fact and it is no wonder the human body is becoming allergic!

Other food additives

There are literally hundreds of different chemicals used in the manufacturing process, to make reconstituted food look and taste better than it really is. It is not proposed to go into them in detail as this subject, by itself, would fill a book. Some examples of food additives are:

Salicylates — Includes a range of chemicals used to flavour tinned, packaged and bottled food artifically.

Tartrazine — This chemical gives rise to a variety of artificial colours such as yellow, orange, blue, red and green and is used in many prepared foods and medications.

Benzoates — Chemicals used in both the artificial preservation and flavouring of a wide range of manufactured foods.

Taken occasionally in foods containing small quantities, these chemicals should not present a health problem. However, because processed foods make up such a large proportion of the average diet; and because virtually all processed foods contain these chemicals; sooner or later the body overloads to a point where the immune system can no longer cope, resulting in allergy sickness and disease.

As far back as the 1930s, some American doctors began to show concern that chemicals could cause illness. However, the onset of the Second World War, followed by the incredible post-war manufacturing boom, rather overshadowed their efforts to prevent, what has now become, a problem of mammoth proportions. The fact that chemicals are making people sick, has recently surfaced again, particularly in the United States. In fact, current thinking in that country is that the growing problem of chemical allergy/intolerance is even more worrying than the growing problem of food intolerance.

At the Kaiser Research Institute, in California, Dr Benjamin Feingold has documented over a hundred cases of sensitivity to artifical flavourings and colourings. These are found in nearly all processed foods such as tinned, packeted, frozen, bottled and cured foods. Dr Feingold says that more than half of all children suffering from hyperactivity, are allergic to certain chemicals in foods. Once these chemicals, namely artificial flavourings, colourings and preservatives are removed from their diet, Dr Feingold has noted a marked improvement in their behaviour. Today, there are several hundred parent-organized branches of the Feingold Association, throughout America, recommending additive-free diets.

Here are some examples of chemicals which are widely used in processed and manufactured foods. Continuous intake of these chemicals will invariably result in toxic overload, leading to degenerative illness:

Benzyl Acetate — Used as a strawberry flavour in many foods. It is also used as a nitrate solvent in the photographic industry.

Amyl Acetate — Used to give ice cream a banana flavour. It is also used in industry as a solvent for oil paint.

Piperonal — Extensively used as a substitute for vanilla flavouring. This chemical is widely used by pest exterminators to kill lice.

Aldehyde — C17 — Used as a flavouring for cherry ice cream and other processed foods. It is also an inflammable chemical used in the manufacture of dyes, plastics and rubber.

Diethyl Glucol — A chemical used as an emulsifier and as a substitute for eggs. It is also used, commercially, as an antifreeze and a paint remover.

Ethyl Acetate — Used to obtain a pineapple flavour. Used in industry as a cleaner for leather and textiles. It has been known to cause severe heart, lung and liver damage to those employed in these industries.

Butyralhyde — Used to provide various nut flavours in processed foods. This chemical is one of the common ingredients used to manufacture rubber cement.

Food additives

These are added to foods for a variety of reasons, among which the shelf-life of the product and its eye-catching appearance are the most important. They are therefore found in many packaged, processed and canned goods. Types of additives include preservatives, colours, flavours, emulsifiers, stabilisers and sweeteners. The following list gives some examples:

Class	Examples
Antioxidants	Butylated hydroxyanisole, butylated hydroxytoluene, various gallate esters, ascorbic acid, tocopherols.
Preservatives, Emulsifiers & stabilisers (structuring agents)	Benzoic acid, sorbic acid, biphenyl-2-o1 Stearoyl tartrate, fatty monoglycerides, aceto, lacto- and citro-glycerides, certain polyglycerol esters, fatty sorbitan esters, cellulose esters, sodium (carboxymethyl) cellulose, agar, alginic acid, carrogeenan, lecithin, Na and Ca caseinate, starch and modified starches.
Sweeteners	Saccharin, cyclamate, peptides
Flour improvers	Benzoyl peroxide
Colours	Various azo dyes, B-carotene
Food acids	Acetic, citric, lactic, malic, succinic acids.

Humectants	Sorbitol
Antifoaming agents	Sodium stearate, silicones.
Glazing agents	Beeswax, spermaceti
Anti-caking agents	Magnesium stearate.
Release agents	Sperm oil, butyl stearate, silicone
Sequestrants	Glycine, salts of ethylenediaminetetra-acetic acid (EDTA).
Propellants	Freons (fluorinated hydrocarbons)
Flavours	Lactones, acetic acid, hydrolyzed protein, esters
Flavour enhancers	Sodium glutamate, inositate and guanylate

This does not include contaminents such as spray residues (fruits, (leafy vegetables), hormones (poultry), ethylene gas (bananas), fumigants (dried fruits, flours) and paraffin (waxed fruits and vegetables).

The following is a more detailed list of some of the most important additives. Because of the widespread distribution of additives, it is generally best to avoid foods presented in packaged, processed or canned form, as labelling of ingredients is not yet standardised in Australia.

Yellow(tartarazine) This is present in many coloured, prepared foods, paticularly cordials, soft drinks, cake mixes, custard powders and medications. It is also present in such items as chewing gum, lollies, macaroni, and other forms of pasta, certain yellow cheeses, yellow ice cream, margarine, yoghurt, coloured breadcrumbs, fish fingers, certain packet or canned soups, mayonnaise and some breakfast cereals. People, sensitive to tartarazine may also react to aspirin.

Red This is present in cordials, soft drinks, lollies, glazed fruits, coloured yoghurt and ice-cream, milk drinks, jellies, bubblegum, medications.

Benzoic Acid   This is widely used as a preservative in soft drinks, cordials, fruit juices, sausage meats, sauces, milk shake syrups, apple cider, bread, chutney, commercial soups and pressed meats.

Sulphur dioxide   This is contained in cordials and soft drinks, dried fruits, pickles, certain wines and ciders. Sulphur dioxide can be removed from dried fruits by boiling.

Monosodium glutamate   This is obtained from the wastes of molasses. It is widely used to enhance the flavour of foods. The following is a list of the type of food in which it is found. Chinese foods, Japanese foods, chicken rolls, fish fingers, beef burgers, packaged chicken curry and rice, nasi goreng, Pork Italienne, gravy mix, meat loaf, seasoning mix, canned sausages, chicken soup cubes, fish pastes and meat spreads, pizza mix, snack biscuits, processed meats and canned soups. Most meat-flavoured products, eg. soy sauce, gravy mix, soups. It occurs naturally in chicken.

Potassium sorbate   This is found in fruit juices and pickles, canned vegetables, cheese spreads, mayonnaise, margarine and certain cheeses.

Hydrocarbon sensitivity

Drs Kenyon and Lewith of Southampton, both eminent clinical ecologists, have studied the effects of hydrocarbon sensitivity.

Hydrocarbon and chemical sensitivity always go hand in hand with food sensitivities. In some patients, the chemical and hydrocarbon sensitivity is more dominant than food sensitivities. In other cases food sensitivities are more important. To date it has been possible to sort out the majority of ecological problems concentrating on foods alone. Sadly this situation is slowly changing and it is becoming necessary to take on the much more difficult task of unravelling patient's hydrocarbon and chemical exposure in order to achieve a reasonable clinical result. The outlook for the future is bleak, as there are no signs that hydrocarbon, pesticide, insecticide, food preservative, food additive and aerosol propellant pollution is on the decrease; if anything, it is very much on the increase. By far the most important sensitivity in this group is that of hydrocarbon sensitivity, specifically sensitivity to gas, petrol and diesel.

What are hydrocarbons? Hydrocarbons contain only the elements of hydrogen and carbon. They occur naturally in petroleum and gas and are used in the manufacture of plastics, solvents, synthetic fibres and synthetic rubbers. Commercial petroleum products, such as petrol, kerosene, aviation fuel and lubricating oils, are derived from mixtures of hydrocarbons. Hydrocarbons are also contained in the gases manufactured from coal and petroleum.

People with hydrocarbon sensitivity will usually feel ill or very tired when exposed to gas, petrol or diesel fumes. They are usually very sensitive to the smell of these fumes, whereas other people would not notice them. Another common symptom is the syndrome termed by American ecologists as 'brain fag'. The person's intellect becomes dulled, his memory is severely affected and often his speech becomes slurred.

Obviously, the hydrocarbon problem is of extreme concern in a world which is so reliant on motor vehicle transportation. However, with care and good management, this problem can be minimised by the sufferer. The obvious things, such as keeping clear of heavy diesel trucks, avoiding self-serve petrol stations and not walking or running near busy roads, can go a long way towards assisting a person, with hydrocarbon sensitivities, to lead a normal life. Because this sensitivity always goes hand in hand with food allergies, often the diagnosis and removal of food allergens will greatly assist the overloaded immune system to cope more efficiently with the remaining chemical/hydrocarbon allergies.

Another major form of hydrocarbon allergy is caused by heating and cooking gas. This can be the most serious of all hydrocarbon problems due to gas appliances, such as fires and cookers, being used in continuous close proximity to the sufferer. Leading American allergist, Dr Theron Randolph, has slated the gas stove as a 'pernicious device'. In the past twenty-five years, he has made three thousand susceptible families switch to something less potentially allergenic. In the case of very sensitive gas allergies, it is necessary to remove completely all gas appliances, pipes and materials regularly exposed to gas, from the home. The obvious choice for these people is electric cooking and heating. The main hydrocarbon derivatives, which cause people problems are paints, varnishes, solvents, cleaning fluids, lighter fluids, aerosol propellants, sponge rubber, plastics, coal tar soaps, detergents, polishes, wax candles, coal fires, air fresheners, deodorants, disinfectants, substances containing phenol and all tinned foods (as the insides of tin cans are coated with phenol), and cosmetics and perfumes.

Fertilizers, insecticides and pesticides

As far back as the 1930s, Dr Albert Rowe, in America, noticed that some of his patients had reactions to apples which had been sprayed with insecticides. He then realized that it was not just apples, but all fruits sprayed with insecticides and pesticides that made some people ill. He coined the term 'multiple fruit sensitivity', and this was probably the first recognition of a problem, which has developed over the past fifty years into the multiple allergy syndrome, which now affects so many people.

People with allergies to pesticides, insecticides and weed killers should ensure that all fruit and vegetables are thoroughly washed before eating. The ideal, of course, is to eat only organically-grown produce, as this has not been contaminated by any of the above, nor by artificial fertilizers. Gardening activities should be approached with great caution, particularly with respect to the various sprays and other chemical substances commonly in use. Even the handling of lawn fertilizers should be considered, as these often contain weed killers. Dr Kenyon reports experiences with patients who had been exposed to pesticides and insecticide. In one case severe progressive brain damage occurred. Another patient became progressively deaf.

An example of the devastating results thought to be caused by exposure to chemicals, is that of Vietnam Veterans, who were exposed to the herbicide Agent Orange. This could be a typical case of an allergenic substance causing illness years after the event. Some feel tired and sick most of the time and have symptoms ranging from brain disorders to major organic disease. Others experience symptoms of fatigue, irritability and irrational behaviour. Yet this product was tested and found to be safe for humans!

Allergies to food, commonplace materials and their odours are symptoms of mysterious chronic illnesses caused by exposure to chemicals.

This observation is a result of the research by a Melbourne neurologist, Dr Malcolm Barr and a former Vietnam serviceman, Mr Michael Boland. Their paper, 'Chemicals, Behaviour and Hyper-Sensitivity: What is the Underlying Biological Mechanism for Food Intolerance?', was written in 1983 and investigated the symptoms of chemical poisoning, especially Agent Orange. Their research was brought to the attention of the public when the *Australian* newspaper (13 May 1983) reported their discussion that

> ... a person exposed to, and thereby made sensitive to, a pesticide might not notice anything wrong immediately but four or five months or a year later, he may be clinically sick and not know why.
>
> As his sensitivity to the pesticide increases, the problem spreads to involve sensitivity to the fumes of his gas range, furnace and water heater, the odour of wall-to-wall carpeting, plastics in the house, the vinyl interior of his car, possibly materials he handles at work — anything from solvents and lubricants to the odour of carbonless copy paper.
>
> Because all these exposures are multiple and daily, this person remains chronically sick, and he and his doctors are confused as to the cause.
>
> As the process spreads, the degree of sensitivity increases — a smaller and smaller amount is sufficient to reactivate the problem.

Allergists have found that certain foods can cause delayed changes in the body. Dr Barr and Mr Boland linked these reactions to tension fatigue syndrome in adults and hyperactivity in children. Their research indicated that the symptoms including headaches, tiredness, depression, confusion and limb and abdominal pains were caused by eating certain foods. Recently some neurological diseases have been found to induce the above syndrome — myalgic encephalomyelitis, subchronic infectious peripheral neuritis and ciguateria poisoning caused by hydrocarbons such as Agent Orange in Vietnam. These diseases are associated with severe allergies to foods like eggs, fish, certain fruits and vegetables, drugs and alcohol. The delayed effects of this hypersensitivity sets it apart from usual allergies.

Their research reinforces the point that there are many people today whose immune systems, bombarded for years with the wrong substances, now cannot cope with substances considered safe. The other point is that, individually, these substances are probably tolerable. The progressive, combined assault of hundreds of chemicals in our daily existence, however, can overload the immune system to such a degree that, sooner or later, allergies to specific substances will develop. These allergies will, quite possibly, be masked in form and difficult to detect.

Drugs

The extraordinary variety of drugs available today, for every conceivable ailment, makes it inevitable that many people, in the course of their lifetime, will become overloaded with the toxic residues of these drugs.

In chapter 3 it was shown that an overloaded immune system can lead to a compounding multiple allergy condition. In the case of too much drug taking, not only will this cause illness, but can also lead to the development of food and other allergies. A system, overloaded with toxins, can start to react to virtually any substance at any time and invariably will unless the individual changes his habits. To quote Ross Horne in his book *The New Health Revolution*:

> The medical system of today is a vast industry orientated to the use of surgery and modern drugs which are 'pushed' upon it by the drug companies. The spectacular success of penicillin and antibiotics years ago, generated a misplaced confidence among doctors and the public alike, which led to ever-increasing drug production and drug dependence.
>
> Aside from improved surgical techniques in treating injuries and congenital defects, orthodox medicine as generally available, is at the end of a blind tunnel. It is simply a defective product being sold at an exorbitant price.

Strong words indeed — but with the harsh ring of truth about them!

Antibiotics

In the endless lists of drugs prescribed by doctors, designed to palliate symptoms rather than cure the cause, antibiotics are amongst the most damaging. Admittedly, in extreme and specific cases, these drugs can work well. Unfortunately, they are prescribed constantly for every type of infection. Often they do no good at all because the body simply does not need or want them. Antibiotics lower the level of immunocompetence due to their depressant effect on the immune system. They should only be taken in extreme cases and preferably not for long periods. It is known that antibiotics knock out useful bacteria in the body, thus upsetting balance and metabolism, which in turn paves the way for allergy illness.

According to Dr D.A. Roe, in his book, *Drug Induced Nutritional Deficiencies,* antibiotics cause malabsorption of nutrients in the small intestine. Pancreatic lipase activity (necessary for digestion of fats) is decreased by antibiotics such as neomycin and streptomycin. The villi are shortened and the intestinal mucosa are infiltrated with inflammatory cells.

Tetracycline, a widely prescribed broad spectrum antibiotic, has been shown to cause liver toxicity, biochemical imbalances in the blood, kidney disease, sensitivity of the skin to light and toxic effects on the foetus such as damage to the teeth and impaired skeletal development.

The contraceptive pill

It is only now, after fifteen to twenty years of constant use, that it is becoming clear that prolonged use of the pill can be very harmful to some women. Indications are that the present epidemic of allergies in the United Kingdom may have been caused by the increase in use of oral contraceptives, during the 1970s. Women taking the pill, over a prolonged period, have been found to have vitamin and mineral deficiencies and other biochemical imbalances. This has resulted in numerous disorders such as impaired immune function and allergies. These facts were published in October 1984 in the *International Clinical Nutrition Review.*

The article went on to say that liver dysfunction was common amongst these women. In addition they suffered from migraines, depression, lowered libido, irritability, anxiety, lethargy, aggression, weight gain, leg cramps, blood vessel disorders and cancer of the breast and cervix. Many of these problems persist after discontinuation of the pill. This is a tragic example of a drug allergy, causing chronic ill health and leading to more serious disease. It indicates that women should try and avoid prolonged use of the pill.

Tap water sensitivity

Tap water sensitivity is not uncommon and is due to the chlorine and fluoride chemicals it contains. People who suspect that they are suffering from food and chemical allergies should not drink water unless a tap filter has been fitted. Alternatively, bottled spring water or distilled water are ideal and probably superior to filtered tap water.

Here are some interesting comments from health researchers on chlorinated water:

Chlorine has so many dangers it should be banned.

Putting chlorine into the water supply is like starting a time bomb. Cancer, heart trouble, premature senility, are conditions attributable to chlorine-treated water supplies.

It has been found that where people drink mountain water, pure and free of chlorine, they tend to live longer.

These are the views of Dr H. Swartz, biological chemist, of Cumberland County College, New Jersey.

We are worrying a lot about chlorine. When chlorine is used to treat water it doesn't disappear. It shows up as part of thousands of new compounds.

Dr Robert Carlson, University of Minnesota.

Chlorine is the greatest crippler and killer of modern times . . . the cause of an unprecedented disease epidemic which includes heart attacks, strokes, senility and sexual impotency.

Dr Joseph Price, chlorine researcher at Saginaur University, Michigan.

There are many other negative comments about chlorinated water by people well respected in various fields of medical research. Sensible people will avoid drinking unfiltered tap water.

Warning comments by a leading Sydney dental surgeon, indicate that fluoridation may be just as sinister as chlorination. He cites warnings, from several highly respected scientific journals, that the population at large is in danger from over-exposure. Apart from the water we drink, fluoride is also getting into our systems from dental fluoridation, medicines, fertilizers, insecticides, pesticides and toothpaste. Aluminium smelters are also responsible for environmental pollution with fluorides. Over-exposure to fluoride, contains all the dangers of chlorine over-exposure. This would tend to make avoidance of unfiltered tap water doubly important.

Soaps and detergents

These contain many chemicals, including formaldehyde (formalin), which is a major source of allergy for most multiple allergy sufferers. Fortunately, there are a number of companies, these days, manufacturing chemically-free soaps and washing powders. However, coal tar soaps and pine-scented soaps should be avoided as these contain hydrocarbons.

Salt

Salt is known to contribute to high blood pressure, heart disease, kidney damage, arthritis and cancer. It is particularly dangerous to multiple allergy sufferers because an excess of salt (sodium chloride) consumes the sodium bicarbonate produced by the pancreas. As described in Chapter 7, production of sodium bicarbonate by the pancreas is extremely important in providing an efficient digestive process. Excessive salt, therefore, can cause pancreatic dysfunction, resulting in acidosis disrupting digestion, thus triggering off food allergies.

According to Professor Ron Wills and his research team, at the University of New South Wales, salt levels in many common processed foods are far too high. After several years of study he is convinced that processed food is the main contributor of salt in most diets — another reason for regular avoidance of processed foods.

Salt can cause irritation to the lining of the stomach, thus affecting the digestive process. When taken on an empty stomach, it robs the stomach lining of water and causes cells to shrivel. Inflammation in the stomach may persist for two weeks after salt has been removed from the diet. Certainly, anything likely to affect digestive efficiency, especially in food allergy sufferers, should be treated with extreme caution.

Aluminium

It is suspected that aluminium cookware may cause problems for the chemically intolerant person, and some countries have limited its use in this regard. Medical analyst, Dr Elizabeth Rees, of California, has found that food not only absorbs aluminium when it is cooked but also when it is wrapped in aluminium foil. Foil-wrapped food keeps longer because the aluminium poisons the bacteria. Major symptoms of aluminium poisoning include throbbing headaches, constipation, hair loss, colic and heartburn. Once again, this is an accumulated overload situation. These symptoms do not happen overnight, but as a result of years of absorption.

Many researchers claim that aluminium is the major cause of the senile dementia known as Alzheimers Disease. This is fast becoming one of the big health problems in Western societies. The symptoms are loss of memory and bizarre behaviour. They have been known to occur from the mid-forties onwards.

The alarming thing is that aluminium is actually added to foods. It is added to processed cheeses to make them melt, and bottled pickles to keep them crisp. In some parts of the world, it is added to drinking water to reduce cloudiness. For a variety of reasons, it is also added to antacids and other pharmaceutical preparations, baking powder, self raising flour, toothpaste, anti-perspirants and non-dairy creamers for tea and coffee.

The purpose of this chapter has been to acquaint the reader, briefly, with the problem of chemical sensitivity. The wide range of symptoms and illness caused by a build up in the system of too many chemicals, over too many years, will cause a multiple allergy condition, incorporating further allergies to foods and other substances.

German researchers have estimated that 50,000 different synthetic substances are circulating in our world today. These are contained in a multitude of foods, drinks, soaps, detergents, cleaning aids, cosmetics, household goods and industrial products — the list is endless. There are more than a hundred million tonnes of chemical substances, currently contained in the food we eat, the water we drink and the air we breathe. Small wonder, as these products continue to be developed at an alarming rate, that Western society is in such dire risk of widespread illness. Already this is beginning to happen and enlightened doctors fear that this backlash to our polluted environment is just the beginning.

10

OTHER ALLERGIES

How important are they?

This book is basically devoted to the concept that, as a result of our modern food and chemical environment, toxins are building up in our bodies, weakening our immune systems and, finally, resulting in multiple allergy conditions and disease.

The preceding chapters have concentrated on discussing food and chemical allergies, and how and why they occur. This chapter will look briefly at the simpler forms of allergies caused by cats, dogs, pollens, etc. People suffering from food and chemical allergies are more susceptible to other forms of allergy due to the poor condition of their immune system. It is most likely therefore, that included in a complex food and chemical allergy condition, will be intolerances to other easily recognizable, allergenic matter.

Pollens

There is no doubt that at certain times of the year, pollens cause many people a distressing array of symptoms. These include hay fever, mucous, red eyes that itch intolerably, overheating and great tiredness. At times, particularly at night, difficulty in breathing may also be experienced.

As far back as 1867, Dr Charles Blackley of Manchester, noted that when pollen was placed on the skin it caused itching and swelling to some people. When pollen is inhaled, it makes contact with the mucous membrane, lining the nose, and absorbs water from the mucous. A substance, not yet identified, dissolves from the pollen and enters the bloodstream through the mucous membrane. It then becomes an antigen which the white cells and antibodies of the immune system would normally destroy.

In the case of an allergic person, the immune system does not destroy the pollen antigen. The presence of the antigen causes the mast cells, which are laden with histamine and other chemicals, to break up and release a flood of histamine to the affected areas. The excessive histamine causes both localised symptoms in the initial areas of contact and general symptoms throughout the body. The former being hay fever, runny nose, etc. and the latter, the accompanying tiredness and lethargy.

Pollens become a problem mainly during spring and also in autumn owing to some plants, chiefly wild grasses, flowering twice a year. As pollens are carried on the wind, it makes little difference whether a sufferer be a country or a city dweller, the allergic reaction will be the same. Fungal spores from plant parasites on grain crops can also trigger allergic reactions in pollen-sensitive people.

Obviously, avoiding exposure to pollens is extremely difficult, apart from staying indoors with the windows closed during the bad times of the year. It is possible, however, for many people to find relief through a programme of desensitisation from a medical allergist. This is given, following a series of skin tests, to ascertain the various types of pollens causing the allergy.

Medication, such as antihistamine tablets and decongestant sprays may be used to seek occasional, temporary relief. These preparations do not cure but simply palliate symptoms to make life a little easier for the sufferer. Beware of prolonged use! In the United States, doctors now suspect that thousands of people have become addicted to nasal sprays. If used too often to constrict blood vessels that have become dilated by histamine, natural constriction ceases to happen efficiently and the nose can become permanently blocked.

While it may not be possible to eliminate symptoms completely, a clean diet and avoidance of allergenic foods and chemicals will assist the immune system to cope better with pollen allergies.

House dust

People who are sensitive to house dust suffer from a form of allergic rhinitis which can cause identical symptoms to those of a pollen allergy. Fortunately, the symptoms usually subside within half an hour once the person has removed himself from the house environment. The normal activities of making beds, dusting, vacuuming, beating mats, etc. tend to bring on the running nose, hay fever and other symptoms which indicate that an allergenic dust has been released into the surrounding air. A sensitive person may find that when he wakes in the morning he has a blocked nose and itchy eyes. In a dusty house he may even wake during the night, wheezing and short of breath. Housewives may have symptoms throughout the day because of constant exposure.

House dust is a composition of cotton, wool fibres, kapok fibres, moulds, human and animal hair, danders (skin flakes), food particles, insect fragments and a variety of substances brought in from outside the house. Although all these materials are to varying degrees, allergenic, the main problem is a living mite — a microscopic, tick-like creature whose main diet is human and animal dander. There are a number of different types of mites; some live in mattresses, whilst others prefer old upholstered furniture. Sensitivity to house dust, therefore, is mainly a sensitivity to the house mite. Treatment of house dust allergy involves removal of the mite and tests to ascertain a course of desensitisation therapy.

Obviously, environmental control is the key to resolving house dust/mite allergy and much can be done to minimise its existence by careful and regular cleaning. In the bedroom, particularly, vacuuming should be done daily and the bed vacuumed at least weekly. Regular exposure of both bed and bedding to sunlight will further retard growth and numbers of the mite. Pets should be excluded from the bedroom and if possible from the rest of the house, as their dander will greatly increase house mite population. Throughout the house regular cleaning is essential. In chronic cases carpets should be replaced by a hard surface with scatter rugs that are aired and beaten daily. Curtains should be of cotton or nylon and washed regularly.

Often, irritation of the nasal mucous membranes has been caused by reaction to an inhaled chemical or an ingested food or chemical. This in turn creates the right climate for a more serious reaction to house dust than might otherwise have occurred. Avoidance of other allergenic substances will help considerably in overcoming house dust sensitivity.

Pets

Allergies to pets can happen at any time without any apparent reason. Dogs and cats are the most likely offenders by virtue of their being in and around the home. However, any animal is potentially allergenic to persons handling it or coming into contact with its usual haunts.

The problem is caused not by the hair of the animal but by powder-fine flakes of skin, known as dander, which are present in the coat of the animal and deposited on carpets, chairs and other places where it may have lain. Individuals may find themselves sensitive to several different species of animals or conversely to a specific breed within the same species. For example, while one person may be allergic to all cats and possibly dogs, another person may be affected only by a specific breed of cat. Children, in particular, are prone to pet allergies due to their tendency to cuddle and play with their pets and, especially, to hold them close to their faces.

The usual symptoms are associated with the respiratory system in the form of hay fever, running nose, etc. but can also occur as a rash at the various points of contact. By far the most alarming symptom can be an asthma attack which may vary in strength from mild to severe. An ongoing, sporadic asthma condition is likely until the cause is identified and removed. In the case of a pet this would mean banishment from the house and may even necessitate finding it a new home. Some relief of symptoms may be gained if the pet is groomed regularly by another person and away from the house. This would have the effect of minimising the number of loose danders which cause the allergy.

Another symptom commonly associated with pet allergies is a rash called *papular urticaria*. In this case, the allergy is not caused by the dander but by the fleas which inhabit the animal. The rash, if scratched, will form bumps and cause the skin to harden and darken. An effective treatment is the application of calamine lotion and avoidance of contact with the animal concerned. Regular applications of flea powder to the pet can minimise the problem.

An uncommon but very nasty condition can result from contact with birds and is called 'bird fanciers lung'. This is caused by a fungus which grows on bird droppings. Spores from the fungus are inhaled, causing the lining of the lung to become inflamed. Untreated, this condition can cause serious and permanent damage. People who work with birds are usually aware of this danger and take steps to avoid its occurrence.

Insects

Allergies to insects can be caused by bites, stings, cast off hairs or scales. By far the most serious are those caused by bee and wasp stings. In the United States they cause more deaths than bites from venomous animals. Most people do not suffer more than minor symptoms but, for the unfortunate few, serious illness and even death can result.

Recent investigations into bee stings have produced some interesting findings. The bee, if brushed away, will leave behind both its sting and a venom sac which continues to pump venom through the barb into the victim. However, if the bee is left to withdraw the sting itself, the injection of venom is much less, resulting in minimal discomfort. Wasps have a different kind of sting mechanism resulting in the victim receiving a full dose every time.

Some people may develop a partial immunity to bee and wasp stings which can increase the more they are stung. Others may become more and more sensitive until they reach a point where they develop a large-scale reaction to stings and can die. We are not,however, talking about the unfortunate person who is stung many times by a swarm of such insects. That situation would cause serious consequences, irrespective of sensitivity.

While I was on army service in Africa, we suffered at times from tsetse fly bites. On crossing from a controlled area into a fly area, we would be assailed by swarms of these insects which in the course of a day's patrolling, would leave one's body covered with hundreds of bites. After a few days, a type of semi-immunity would develop which seemed to result in fewer bites and less discomfort.

Sometimes, however, an individual soldier would not develop this immunity. Instead, his sensitivity would increase causing sickness and fever and finally lead to his evacuation. This is an example of how some people can build up tolerance by repeated exposure, whilst others become more sensitised.

The usual reaction to stings by a non-allergic person is one of soreness and localised swelling which subsides after a while. Reactions by the allergic person, however, can involve swelling in other parts of the body, aching joints, a general rash and a sensation of dizziness and nausea. Severe reactions, caused by the sudden release of enormous quantities of histamine, can drastically lower the blood pressure, affect the heart and result in unconsciousness and even death. An immediate injection of adrenalin is necessary in these cases if the victim is to survive.

Other insects such as mosquitoes, midges and horseflies can cause reactions by their bite, resulting in a discomforting array of symptoms that are rarely dangerous. One important fact emerging in recent years is that people prone to simple allergies such as insects, pollen, etc. often have food and chemical allergies as well. When this is the case their reaction is invariably more severe than that of the allergy-free person. This indicates that an immune system, free from the stresses of an overloaded toxic condition, is better equipped to cope with all types of allergies, regardless of their origin.

Occupational allergies

As most people spend nearly half their waking lives at work, their work environment will be a major source of contact with possible allergenic substances.

Mention has been made in previous chapters of people eating wheat flour products and suffering allergy symtoms. Allergy problems can also result from the handling of wheat by farm workers and contact with wheat flour, by mill and bakery workers. In the former case, it is thought that concentrations of grain dust and fungal spores affected farm workers. A study of sixteen farmers in the United Kingdom revealed that one quarter of farm workers in dusty, grain storage areas suffered from asthma. Sensitisation usually occurred after several years although sometimes it took as long as ten to twelve years for the symptoms to develop. In the case of millers and bakers it was found that reactions were due to a mite known as *acarus farinae* or more commonly, as the 'flour mite'. Allergy to this mite causes severe skin reaction. Further reaction to flour causing urticaria as well as nasal and bronchial symptoms, is thought to be due to the various chemicals added to the flour during the milling process to whiten it and preserve it.

Allergies due to contact with work-related substances are plentiful. Over eight hundred substances have been listed as contact allergens. They include rubber, dyes, paints, cosmetics, medicines, epoxy resins, chrome and nickel. In a study of workers, exposed to proteolytic enzymes, in a Sydney soap factory, it was found that some workers developed rashes and severe itching of the skin. Other symptoms such as itchy eyes, swollen runny nose and hay fever persisted. Some also developed a dry, hacking cough and others, asthma. Enzymes in the soap industry have long been known to cause allergies. As a result, protective measures have reduced the problem, but the fact remains that some people cannot work in that industry. Researchers at Sydney University have found that proteolytic enzymes occurring naturally in grass thatch cause chronic lung disorders amongst New Guinea tribesmen.

Other forms of contact allergy are to be found constantly throughout commerce and industry. Allergies to printers' ink, coffee dust, platinum salts (used in the photographic industry) and pharmaceutical drugs are just some further examples of this wide-ranging problem.

The more a person becomes sensitised to an allergenic substance, the more likely he is to develop further allergies as the immune system begins to break down. All allergies, therefore, should be taken seriously by the sufferer with strict avoidance of known allergenic substances being the cardinal rule.

ALLERGY TESTING

Facts and fallacies

Conventional medicine has generally not been successful in the diagnosis and treatment of allergies. Limited success has been achieved with airborne and home-related causes such as pollens, dust, house mites and pets. Because of this, specialists have continued to use similar methods in attempts to detect food and chemical sensitivities. The results have invariably been poor with testing proving to be inaccurate and treatment ineffective.

Why then do doctors persist in using medical techniques that do not do the job? The answer is simple. In this age of the much publicised 'wonder drug', people have come to expect quick diagnosis and treatment. Doctors, as well as patients, have fallen into the convenient trap of looking to drugs and chemicals for prompt results. It is faster and simpler to buy an allergy test kit from a drug manufacturer and use it on a patient, than to persist over a period of time with observation and deduction. If the test kit does not work the doctor explains that he cannot do more until medical science produces a better one. This reliance on manufactured preparations has tended to work against allergy sufferers, and it is only comparatively recently that alternative clinical methods of diagnosis have begun to emerge.

Before we move onto more recent developments, we should take a look at some of the tests, currently available, and their relative effectiveness.

Conventional allergy tests

Prick Test

Extracts of well-known allergens such as pollen, house mite or cat dander, are manufactured by drug companies for use in a variety of tests, to ascertain which substances are allergenic to a specific individual.

A simple test is carried out, by placing a drop of the extract on the skin of the forearm and gently pricking it into the upper layer of skin. Up to twenty, or more, of these pricks, each with a different substance, can be carried out in one visit to the allergist. If you are sensitive to a substance, the spot will swell slightly and become red within about fifteen minutes. This does not mean, however, that you are allergic to that substance, simply that, were you exposed to it often enough, or for long enough, you might become allergic to it. It could also mean that you were once allergic to it but, for some reason, are no longer. Even a positive result is far from conclusive and, at best, gives a vague indication only. Nevertheless, this form of testing has had some success in diagnosis and treatment of the airborne, or household, type of allergy. It is also quite often used to test for food allergies and, for this purpose, it is totally unreliable.

Because allergies affect the immune system, it is possible, by examining its structure, to see why skin tests do not detect food and chemical allergies. In Chapter 3 mention was made of antibodies which the immune system manufactures in order to destroy antigens. These antibodies are known medically as 'immunoglobulins', of which there are five main types, IgE, IgD, IgG, IgM and IgA.

IgE is bound to mast cells and resides mainly in the skin mucosa, where it is responsible for contact reactions and allergic manifestations, such as urticaria. In the case of an allergy reaction, the IgE, when confronted with an antigen such as pollen, does not destroy it. Instead, the antigen causes the mast cell, to which the IgE is attached, to break up and release a flood of histamine, which in turn gives rise to the allergy symptoms. IgD is thought to initiate IgE production. IgG and IgM antibodies are found mainly in the blood. It is their job to travel the body and ward off infection by dealing swiftly with invading antigens such as foreign bacteria. In addition IgM acts as a rallying point for a number of IgGs to bind together and form a stronger defence mechanism.

IgA is found mainly in the gut and is produced by the gastro-intestinal cells. It acts in a similar way to IgG and IgM, but, instead of patrolling the body, it remains *in situ* in the stomach and intestine. There, it is ready to attack harmful substances brought in to the body by the process of eating and drinking.

Skin testing, therefore, is likely to stimulate only the IgE system. The systems most likely to be involved with food and ingested chemicals, namely the IgG, IgM and IgA systems, cannot be reached through skin testing. Consequently, skin testing can stimulate the IgE system to produce an allergic response to pollens and house mites, but will fail to stimulate other antibodies to react to food substances.

Patch Test

This is a similar test to the skin prick test except it is used only to ascertain allergies to the skin. In this respect, it is a sensible exercise and has a reasonable success rate. It is effected by a piece of the allergenic substance being taped, or placed, onto the skin for a period of twenty-four hours. Subsequent reaction will then indicate whether an allergy to the substance exists.

Intradermal Test

This is really an extension of the skin prick test. Instead of pricking the substance into the skin, it is injected into the outer layers of skin, on the outside of the upper arm or the inside of the forearm. It is felt that in some cases, this method may give a better response than the prick test, however, both tests are very similar in their application. If the reaction is positive, a small red swelling will show within ten minutes. Sometimes, however, a delayed reaction may occur several hours later.

The intradermal skin test stimulates the IgE system, found mainly in the skin, to react to allergens which normally enter the body through the skin. It relies upon histamine, produced by the IgE mast cells, to produce the red swelling which indicates an allergic response. Clinical ecologists have found that IgE is often not present with IgG, IgM and IgA in food allergies and, therefore, a skin test, which is IgE mediated, used to isolate an immune disturbance that is IgG or IgM mediated, will give an inaccurate result. Skin testing, therefore is of limited use and it is notoriously inaccurate for food testing but it can help to detect some allergies in certain people.

Sublingual Test

The test substance, in solution, is placed under the tongue. This test is sometimes used by doctors in an attempt to identify suspect food allergies. It is not effective for similar reasons to those that render skin tests ineffective. However, whereas the skin test is IgE mediated, the sublingual test is, probably, IgA mediated, whilst the food allergies being tested, are often IgG or IgM mediated. This is another example of testing which does not contact the right immunoglobulin to enable an accurate result to be achieved.

Cytotoxic Testing

The word 'cytotoxic' is derived from the Greek word *CYTO* which means 'cells' and 'toxic' which means 'poisonous'. A cytotoxic reaction, therefore, is one that effects the cells, or more specifically, the white blood cells.

It is now possible to observe the effect some food substances have on the white blood cells, under a microscope. This is due to work done by an American, Dr Arthur Black, in the 1950s. In Australia, there are about a hundred foods that can be tested in this manner which involves taking a sample of blood and submitting it for laboratory analysis.

The test is unique because, as not all allergic reactions are mediated by antibodies, ecological problems, in the form of non-immunological allergies, can sometimes be detected. This method can also discover reactions to substances that, otherwise, produce no symptoms — that is, none that are yet detectable by the individual — even though they may already be damaging the body. This application can be useful in the detection of masked food allergies, which often provoke stray cravings, without identifiable after-effects. Some chemical intolerances can also be detected with this method.

Unfortunately, cytotoxic food testing, like most other allergy tests, does not always produce accurate, or complete, results. It requires only one major allergen to remain undiscovered, for the ongoing and distressing effects of allergy illness to continue.

RAST Test (Radio-allergo sorbant assay)

This is a fairly recent immunological test which is not solely reliant on the response of only one immunoglobulin, such as with the skin test. The antigen to be tested is fixed to small particles and labelled by a radioactive process. It is then mixed with a specimen of the individual's blood serum in order to stimulate a response from one of the immunoglobulins. The presence of immunoglobulins, other than IgE, provides scope for a more accurate allergic response to the antigen. The blood serum is washed and radioactively counted to find out which immunoglobulin has reacted with the antigen, thus indicating whether an allergic reaction has taken place.

This test is certainly an improvement on skin testing as it has been found to be useful in detecting food and chemical allergies. However, it does not always produce accurate answers and so is of limited use compared with other forms of testing which are now available.

Blood sugar

American allergists constantly monitor blood sugar to pick up allergy reactions. After a test food is eaten, they will take blood samples at regular intervals, to ascertain whether an abnormal peak has occurred and at what point this has happened. They have found that allergy reactions to carbohydrates will peak at thirty minutes, fruits at forty-five minutes and most other foods at about sixty minutes, after eating.

This is a particularly useful diagnostic indicator and it is a great pity that doctors in Australia are not more conversant with this method.

Clinical ecology

Clinical ecologists make use of skin tests, where appropriate, but do not rely on them to reveal food and chemical allergies. They realize that there is much still not understood about allergies and their effect on the immune system. Studies of ecological illness have shown that an increasing number of people throughout the Western world, are developing multiple allergies to their diet and chemical environment. These ecology-caused illnesses do not produce the normally accepted responses within the immune system. Therefore, attempts to stimulate the appropriate immunoglobulin, as in standard allergy tests, will not give an indication of allergy to a particular substance. It is apparent, at this stage, that medical science is not in a position to explain why people become sensitive to various foods and/or chemicals, and the mechanism of this sensitivity.

For this reason, clinical ecologists have had to develop other techniques of diagnosing food and chemical sensitivities in the increasing numbers of people presenting this problem. Bearing in mind that many conditions involve multiple masked allergies, it is no easy task to commence the painstaking business of unravelling them. Most dedicated clinical ecologists tend to use a combination approach. They ascertain what they can with conventional testing and invariably, as this produces limited results, they then look to other methods, as well as a careful and detailed study of the individual's diet and chemical environment. Unfortunately, very few doctors are willing to become involved in this difficult field of medicine. The attractions for solving people's health problems, with prescribed drugs, is obvious. The trouble is that this approach often does not work, and the patient lingers on in a twilight world of continuous illness palliated by drugs but never cured, with the quality of his life drastically reduced.

Among the alternative diagnostic techniques evolved by clinical ecologists, is the elimination of allergenic foods by dietary control. This is then followed by reintroduction of suspect foods, over a period of time, with careful notice being taken of possible reactions. The process itself is tedious but simple. Where there is no interested doctor accessible, the individual can carry out this process himself. It does, however, require sound management and self discipline.

Alternative diagnostic techniques have been refined in America, in recent years. According to Dr Carl Ebnother, director of the Centre for Orthomolecular Medicine in California, tests can now be done for 150 food allergies. Dr Ebnother says that the average person today is allergic to 25 foods. If this is the case, then it is no wonder there are so many health problems in America and similar countries, such as Australia. It indicates that most people are suffering from some form of ill health, due to an overload of allergenic toxins.

Testing by use of the Elimination Diet and the reintroduction of foods

Exhaustive investigation of food allergies over the past few years, has shown that some foods are relatively safe for most people. These are known as 'hypo-allergenic foods' and consist of lamb, rice, potatoes, lettuce, parsley and pears.

The principle of the elimination diet is to exclude all foods, except hypo-allergenic foods, for at least two weeks. During this time, the only liquid allowed is spring water, filtered tap water or distilled water. The foods should be cooked in such a way that no other agents, such as butter or oil, are used. In other words, the meat should be grilled and the vegetables steamed, or eaten raw. It is absolutely essential not to use salt, herbs, condiments, garnishes or any additive, which would, in effect, introduce further foods, thus destroying the hypo-allergenic safety of the diet.

In some extreme cases, such as my own, there may be an allergy to rice and/or potatoes as well. Therefore, for the first four days of the elimination diet, these foods should be excluded. On the fifth day introduce one of the foods and, if no reaction, introduce the other twenty-four hours later. Stay on the six basic foods for the remainder of the fortnight, or longer if possible, before further food testing.

Initially it is hard on the taste buds, and those with masked food allergies will suffer from cravings for their favourite foods. However, perseverence is worthwhile, because at the end of two weeks, allergic people following this plan will generally feel better than they have felt in a long time. The reason is that the body has a chance to rid itself of all the accumulated toxins that have been overloading the system for so long. In addition, the safe foods do not leave allergy-caused toxins behind, resulting in the body being clean and free.

It is absolutely essential that nothing else be taken, or eaten, during this time. Medication should be avoided if possible, so consult your doctor first if necessary. In some cases you will feel so good after a few days, that you may be able to reduce some forms of medication, under your doctor's supervision, or even dispense with it entirely. Vitamin and mineral supplements are not necessary during this time. They will simply negate the whole exercise by introducing toxic substances in the form of fillers, flavourings and colourings.

After a few days, you will find that it is not necessary to think in terms of three meals per day. It will be easier to miss meals and, perhaps, fast for a day or two as your body ceases to crave for allergenic foods. Remember, it is not necessary to eat much at all during the two weeks. The basic elimination diet is simply an alternative to direct fasting for people who feel that they must eat something. The more load you can take off the body during this time, the better.

After two weeks, the challenging process begins. By this time, the body has eliminated accumulated toxins and allergenic matter. Thus, if an allergenic food is now introduced, the resultant reaction can be attributed to that food, without the fear of other foods masking the reaction. As the whole purpose of the exercise is to detect the foods that are making you ill, the first thing to do is to start introducing, on a daily basis, foods known to be allergenic. (Refer to the list on the following page.)

Only one new food should be tried each day and this should be eaten, if possible, as a complete meal, or alternatively, eaten with food to which you are not allergic. It is important not to eat composite foods, because if a reaction occurs, you will not know which food has caused it. A diary should be kept, noting the symptoms, how long after eating they occurred, how long they lasted and grading them on a scale of one to five for severity. This will be of considerable assistance later, in deciding the foods to which you are most allergic.

Symptoms may vary considerably. As the body is now clean, they will be easily recognizable and may develop almost immediately, or take up to twenty-four hours. Normally, however, they should become obvious, within the first two hours, after eating the food.

Elimination Diet

Suggested order of food testing

Day	Food	Day	Food
1	Cabbage	16	Onions
2	Tomatoes (well washed)	17	Apples (well washed)
3	Decaffeinated coffee	18	Chicken
4	Beef	19	Grapes (well washed)
5	Carrots	20	Chocolate
6	Oranges	21	Pork
7	Eggs	22	Olive oil (test with a safe food)
8	Milk	23	Tap water
9	Peas	24	Butter
10	Beans	25	Mushrooms
11	Wheat (as a pure wheat cereal)	26	Nuts
12	Cane sugar (labelled cane sugar)	27	Cheese
13	Tea	28	Pineapple
14	Bananas	29	Instant coffee
15	Fish (not shell fish)	30	White sugar

All food must be fresh. Tinned, processed or frozen food is completely unsuitable.

Symptoms to watch out for are headache, accelerated heart beat, fuzzy feeling in the head, hay fever, catarrh, blocked nose, heaviness, lethargy, muscular aching, bloatedness, swollen abdomen, irritability, depression, poor concentration and any other discomfort experienced after eating.

Once symptoms have shown themselves, and been duly recorded, it is possible to reduce their severity, or even stop them, by taking a mixture of one part potassium bicarbonate, to two parts sodium bicarbonate, in a glass of water. The sodium bicarbonate helps neutralize the metabolic acidosis, occurring during the food reaction, whilst the potassium bicarbonate acts as a mild laxative, to hasten the allergens through the system.

Keeping records of reactions is important because, after many weeks of testing, it is then possible to assess when foods should be retested. Retesting is an essential part of the reintroduction process. Many food allergies are 'cyclic' and, after a period of abstinence, which may vary from three to twelve months, it may be possible to eat such foods again. Other food allergies are 'fixed' and no amount of abstinence will allow these foods to be eaten without an allergy reaction occurring.

It is important to understand that the longer the period of total abstinence from the food, the more likely the immune system is to recover and build up a tolerance to that food. Even so, repeated ingestion can awaken the old allergy and the problem recommences. Always to treat foods, that have been previously allergenic, with care and, certainly, never eat them again on a daily basis. At the first sign of symptoms reappearing, the food should not be eaten for a further period of three months, followed by retesting.

Once the initial reintroduction and testing of foods has been completed, a dietary programme should be set up to ensure that safe foods are eaten on a rotational basis. Remember that you are in this position because your immune system has partly broken down. To assist it to build back to full function, allergenic foods must be strictly avoided, and other foods should be spaced out to avoid further allergies developing. The prognosis is excellent, once allergies have been detected and sound management of diet commenced. With the cessation of daily bombardment by allergens, the immune system will rebuild itself, so that after a period of twelve months, providing no permanent damage has been done, a return to full health can be expected. However, caution must always be exercised, in the future, with foods that you have been allergic to in the past.

During the recovery period, and forever after, it is vital to avoid junk food. Intake of refined carbohydrates should virtually cease. One can spoil oneself on occasions, but these should always be the exceptions, never the rule. In particular, processed foods with all their additive chemicals, should be avoided as these will tend to overload the immune system and restart the allergy process. In other words, a clean diet of unprocessed, wholesome, non allergenic foods is essential to maintain good health.

Common allergenic foods

Milk and dairy products Butter

Cheese

Cream

Yoghurt

Grain products All breakfast cereals

Wheat (includes bread, cakes, scones, all flour products)

Oats

Rice

Rye

Barley

Maize

Eggs

Fish (especially shellfish)

Sugar

Yeast (included in bread, alcohol, mushrooms, tinned foods)

Citrus fruits (especially oranges)

Tomatoes (and other members of deadly nightshade group)

Mushrooms (contain yeast)

Pork (including ham and bacon)

Chocolate, cocoa, etc.

Coffee

Tea

Nuts (especially peanuts)

Soya   Beans

       Milk

       Tofu

Tinned food (chemicals — no enzymes)

Frozen food (chemicals)

Alcohol (especially red wine and beer)

Tap water (chemicals)

Testing by use of the fast and reintroduction of foods

This is a similar process to that just described, the difference being that, instead of using the two-week elimination diet to cleanse the body, a fast is undertaken for a period of five days. During this time, nothing is eaten and this must be strictly enforced. The only substance that may be ingested, throughout the five day period, is spring water, preferably, or if unavailable, filtered tap water. Distilled water is also very useful, but should not be taken if it has been previously stored in a plastic container. Remember, plastic is a hydrocarbon derivative and most food allergy sufferers are also allergic to chemicals — hydrocarbon being a principal offender.

The advantage of the fast is that it is completely allergy free. During the five days, the body dispels the accumulated allergens and toxic rubbish that have been overloading it for years. It is a relatively quick, and highly efficient, method of cleaning out the body.

The disadvantages are that you get very hungry and also suffer from withdrawal symptoms, due to masked allergies. For the first three days many people will need encouragement to keep going, as the withdrawal symptoms invariably get worse. By the fourth day these have usually subsided, and by the fifth day most people experience a marked improvement in their sense of well-being.

Fasting is not examined in great detail now, as a chapter has been devoted to it later in this book. Suffice it to say, that fasting, and reintroduction of foods, is one of the methods that consistently proves itself in the detection of masked food allergies.

It is important to remember that the two methods just described, are practical tests, done over a period of weeks, preferably under the supervision of a medical practitioner trained in clinical ecology. They are far superior to the allergy tests that can be given in fifteen minutes, by any general practitioner, and which, for reasons already explained, do not work.

The elimination diet, the fast, and practical food testing, by the reintroduction of foods, are the most important breakthroughs in recent years. Until recently, they have been the only successful methods, devised to enable people to recover from the crushing effects of masked allergy illness. It is a pity that in Australia today, the general practitioner is steadfastly refusing to use these methods, resulting in needless suffering to many thousands of people.

Looking back over my own experiences during the past few years, it is easy now to understand why earlier dietary attempts at solving my health problems failed. At that time the whole concept appeared vague and indeterminate. The medical profession knew nothing of masked allergies and I, like most people, put my faith, solely in doctors. After all, if they could not cure me, who could? I was full of despair and constantly exhausted by the daily grind of working hard and, at the same time, coping with my illness. I understood nothing of masked allergies and withdrawal symptoms, or how it was possible to be addicted to several foods and substances without knowing it. I knew nothing of ecological illnesses, or their effect on the human body. I had only the vaguest notion of the immune system and knew virtually nothing about the major organs, particularly the pancreas. In fact, I was the classic example of the average person, who is kept in ignorance about the workings of his own body. Confused about my health and unable to find help, I did not want to admit, even to myself, just how sick I was becoming. What good would it have done anyway?

Electrical testing — Vega Therapy

Probably the most exciting development to have evolved in recent years, is an electronic procedure for detecting all allergy conditions. It is of particular use in revealing masked allergies and is safe, fast, simple and efficient. It is called Vega Therapy and uses electronic equipment, manufactured by the VEGA Grieshaber Corporation, of West Germany.

In the early part of this century, Dr Hamish Boyd, of Glasgow, noted that if a substance was brought into series in an electrical circuit, to which the patient was connected, a change in skin impedance was produced. Boyd's discovery was the subject of a government inquiry, but nothing further came of it. Then, in the 1950s, a German doctor, Reinholdt Voll, developed Boyd's idea and, with the help of electronic equipment, evolved a useful, but highly complex, technique to diagnose disease. More recently, Dr Helmut Schimmel, also of West Germany, simplified Dr Voll's technique and improved the cumbersome equipment to that of a small portable, electronic unit, known as the VEGATEST.

Dr Julian Kenyon, of Britain, has developed a highly efficient technique for diagnosing allergies, using the VEGATEST equipment. He describes his technique as follows:

The observed fact of changes in skin impedance, provides a useful technique in the field of food and chemical sensitivity. Therefore, the technique can be used for allergy testing. In practice, a point is taken on the fingers or toes, (these are sites where major electrical exchanges happen, between the body and its environment, this being largely due to the geometry of fingers and toes, in that they are relatively pointed and, therefore, charge accumulation occurs at the tips of the digits). A relevant acupuncture point is chosen, although it doesn't appear important to choose any specific point. One by one, the suspected allergens are introduced into the circuit, and each time a new measurement is made. Any substance which causes a drop in measured resistance, is labelled as allergic, or more correctly, in the field of clinical ecology, as 'sensitive', as far as the patient is concerned. In clinical practice, the techniques give the right answer nine times out of ten, which represents a better success rate, than the most successful method for diagnosis of food and chemical sensitivities, available so far, that of Cytotoxic testing. Immunological tests such as the RAST test, (IgE test) for diagnosis of food and chemical sensitivity; are notoriously inaccurate. Those doctors who adhere to these tests in a stubborn fashion, do not appear to be aware, that the results from such tests are often irrelevant, to the patient. The inaccuracy of skin testing, particularly for foods, has been amply demonstrated, by many studies carried out in America, as early as the 1950s.

The existence of electrical changes around biological structures, and their importance both in health and disease, is slowly becoming recognized, but in order for this important study to develop further, closer co-operation between physicists, electronic engineers and medical scientists will have to come about.

The important work done in this field is described by Dr Ion Dumitrescu, of Rumania, in his book, *Electrographic Imaging in Medicine and Biology*. To date, Dr Kenyon has trained several hundred doctors, in the United Kingdom, in the use of the VEGATEST for allergy diagnosis.. He has also lectured throughout Europe, America and Asia, to several thousand more doctors who are genuinely interested in helping patients overcome multiple allergy illness.

A great advantage of the VEGATEST method is that it can detect any allergic substance, whether it be food, chemical, airborne, environmental or whatever. Not only that, but it can also measure the degree of sensitivity — something which no other allergy test can do.

Diagnosis is the key to allergy illness. Once the food/chemical substances have been detected, avoidance will usually enable the patient to recover quickly. It is absolutely impossible to comprehend, when you are staggering through life under the deadly weight of allergy illness, just how wonderful and alert it is possible to feel, within a few short days or weeks, of successful diagnosis and avoidance. Diagnosis is the key and, in Australia, for most people, it is a very elusive key indeed!

The good news for chemical allergy sufferers is that, once diagnosis is achieved, it is possible for clinical ecologists, such as Dr Kenyon, to switch off some allergies, by means of desensitising drops or injections. However, this method is not very successful for treating food allergies. Avoidance is by far the best. This subject will be discussed in detail in Chapter 13.

Some other practical food tests, which can be put to good use by suspected sufferers, are the pulse test, the kinesiology test and the urine test.

The Pulse Test

Dr Arthur Coca, an American clinical ecologist, has devised a test known as the pulse test. He discovered that your pulse rate goes up after you have eaten, or inhaled, an allergenic substance. However, certain rules must be obeyed in order for the test to be successful. These are:

Stop smoking. Tobacco is a major allergen and distorts the pulse rate.

Test your pulse throughout the day and keep a record. If the difference between your highest and lowest pulse rate is more than 12 beats, then you are allergic to something you ate that day.

Write down each food you eat at each meal.

When testing, eat a portion of a single food and then take your pulse every fifteen to thirty minutes, for an hour and a half afterwards. If your pulse rises above 84 beats per minute, into the high 80s or 90s, this is indicative of an allergic reaction.

It is essential to wait until the pulse rate returns to normal before further testing. This may take one to several hours. A rise of 6 beats or more, generally indicates an allergic reaction. Inhalants may show a smaller rise and yet still be allergic. If your pulse differential remains high, no matter what you eat, then you are allergic to most things that you are eating — or to something you are constantly inhaling.

The pulse test is a useful self-help method of detecting food/chemical allergies. It does not pick up all maladaptive reactions.

The Kinesiology Test

This is a simple method for detecting some food/chemical sensitivities and has been known for centuries. It involves placing substances under the tongue and testing their effect on muscle strength.

Here's how you do it: First test your muscle strength under normal circumstances by holding your arm out in front of you palm down. Have someone then exert pressure on your arm and together work out your level of resistance. Next, chew a small mouthful of the suspect food and place it under the tongue. Do not swallow it. Leave the food under the tongue and again, test your level of resistance. If you find your arm weaker than before, it is very likely that you are allergic to the food. Often, this test will show a marked weakness, indicating food allergy. Once this has occurred, spit out the food and proceed to test the next one.

Although this test is not sufficiently accurate for minor allergies, it can certainly be a good indicator for major ones. It is best used with simple substances, such as wheat flour, sugar, milk, coffee, etc.

Urine Test

This is a useful test which can be carried out with the use of a long wave, ultra violet light. These are not expensive and can be obtained through a pharmacy or medical supply company.

First test your urine, before eating, to see if it is normal, by shining the light downwards at a 45 degree angle on to a test tube, three quarters full. If normal, it will range from a straw colour, through to a clear colour. Having checked this, now proceed to eat a reasonable amount of a single food to be tested.

After three hours have lapsed, again take a urine sample and shine the ultra violet light downwards, onto the test tube at a 45 degree angle. If the food is allergenic, the urine in the test tube will show blue in colour. The shade can range from light to dark, indicating the intensity of the reaction. Sometimes, the colour will show as a pink, through to a deep red. This indicates porphyria (toxic mercury level) which is also linked to an allergic reaction.

FASTING AND FOOD TESTING

Anyone can do it

The fast would probably have been first used by our ancient predecessors in their early attempts to treat illness. After all, it makes sense to give the body a rest from the daily rigours of the digestive processes.

The benefits of fasting are without dispute. Throughout the known history of every civilization, race and culture, fasting has featured significantly for both religious and health reasons. Even religious fasts were based on sound physiological principles. The ancients knew that it was difficult to think good thoughts when the body was overloaded with toxic rubbish.

In animals, the abstinence process is instinctive. As a result, not only will the animal fast and rest, when it is sick or injured, but it will also avoid eating any food which may be harmful to it. This is not quite the case in domesticated animals, as they can acquire the bad habits of their owners, if given the chance. Unfortunately, human beings (especially those living in modern industrialised societies), have had their basic sensory mechanisms blunted by the unnatural processing and extraordinary diversity of the Western diet. As a result, we are no longer, instinctively, able to recognize what is good for us and what is not. If we could, there would be very little sickness in the world today and, certainly, the ever increasing problem of masked multiple allergies would simply not exist.

Many people, these days, experience toxic overload, to some degree, due to:

Habitually eating more food than is required for the body's needs.

Poor quality, processed foods, which impose a strain on the digestive and assimilative functions of the body.

Lack of exercise, which reduces the detoxifying capacities of the liver and kidneys, and affects the excretory efficiency of the bowels and bladder.

Allergy sufferers have these problems further aggravated by the additional toxins permanently present in their bodies, as a result of allergenic substances. A primary cause of allergy illness is food allergy. Obviously, if a sufferer stops eating he will feel better.

The fasting process

When we eat, or engage in physical acitivity, our food must be broken down into component nutrients and then built up into cellular tissue, or energy supply. The residue must be collected and eliminated. If allergenic food is constantly ingested, toxicity will accumulate, resulting in discomfort and illness. This is further exacerbated by too much food, containing excessive, unusable matter. Fasting, therefore, allows the continuation of the brief cleansing period that takes place during sleep. It is important during a fast to rest as much as possible, so that all available bodily energy can be directed to the cleansing process. With no food in the gastrointestinal tract and no tension in the muscular or nervous systems, this can take place with maximum efficiency.

During the fasting process, the body lives on its stored reserves. These are contained in every cell and every organ, in the form of glycogen in the liver, protein in the blood and lymph, stored fat, (even in thin people) and assorted food elements in the bone marrow and glands.

One of the incredible things about the fasting process, is that in a few short days, the accumulated toxicity from years of illness can be obliterated due to the body's incredible capacity to recover. The temporary suspension of its digestive and eliminative labours, increases this capacity greatly. In no time at all the body is relatively clean, thus allowing food testing to commence.

The cleansing action taking place during the fast results in the toxic residues being eliminated in many different ways. Bowel and bladder movements are considerably reduced. Contrary to popular belief, it is not necessary to drink copious quantities of water. However, a litre of pure water per day, should be the average intake, with more if necessary, depending on the state of health of the individual. Elimination through the ears, nose, mouth and pores will continue constantly throughout the fast until all toxins are consumed. The tongue, in particular, will take on a concentrated 'furriness' and this is a good indication that toxic elimination is working properly. After a few days, this will pass.

It is important to understand that a fast is the quickest way to clean the body and recover from an overloaded, toxic, allergy-inducing state. This means having no food at all if it is to work effectively, in the shortest possible time. Partial fasts, such as the grape diet, are not really fasts at all and, although a single food diet will facilitate valuable cleansing, it will obviously take longer to achieve. The body cannot metabolise nutritional intake and, at the same time, effectively break down stored reserves.

When you consider that, in the course of a normal day's food intake, the pancreas produces three quarters of a litre of digestive juices, and the liver about a litre of bile, it is easy to see why a fast would be beneficial to these vital organs and, at the same time would release energy for toxin elimination.

It is important to consult your doctor before commencing a fast. Normally this is a safe process, but some medical conditions may need careful monitoring.

Preparing for the fast

A reduced diet, containing fruit and vegetable juices, is of great value in preparing the body for a fast. This will assist the stomach to prepare for less food and finally no food. The fatty tissues will also be stimulated into readiness to give up some of their bulk and stored toxicity. In preparation for the five day fast, (followed by reintroduction of foods) eating should be scaled down during the week prior, with diet for the last three days, consisting of fruits, salads and juices.

One method of scaling down eating, before commencing a fast, is, simply, to cut back to two meals per day, for a few days, ensuring they become smaller and lighter as each day goes by. The day before the fast, one light meal only, should be eaten.

When to fast

For the multiple allergy sufferer, the fast is the first step to recovery and good health. Within a few days the body is cleansed of allergenic substances, and you can feel free of symptoms perhaps for the first time in years. Only when the body is symptom-free can you get down to the all important task of finding out which foods and substances have been making you sick.

Obviously, the best time for an allergy sufferer to fast is straight away. Don't waste time. Start lightening your meals and cutting back now. If it may mean some time off work, then take it. This is an investment in your whole future and well-being. Do not attempt to do your fast and work as well. It is better to use the elimination diet, which takes longer, but should allow most sufferers to be relatively symptom-free, after a fortnight. Fasting needs rest. The two go hand in hand and should never be separated. Whilst the elimination diet is useful for most people, fasting is the ideal, and should be undertaken, either in preference to the elimination diet, or in addition to it, whenever possible.

If you are unwell, as a result of undiagnosed food and chemical allergies, the symptoms, as we have seen, can be in almost any form. Subject to your doctor's approval, it is not necessary to wait for recovery from cold or flu. In fact, an ideal time to commence a fast is when the body's temperature has risen a few degrees, when a state of crisis prevails. Feverishness, headache, muscular pains and general debility are some of the indications. It is then that the body is working hard to throw off the overload of toxins which, in the case of masked allergies, it can never do. Suppression of these symptoms by drugs will simply compound the allergy problem into more deeply-rooted, chronic illness.

The five-day fast

The five-day fast is the most efficient method of ridding the body of stored allergens, thus paving the way for a steady recovery. At the commencement of the fast, a good dose of epsom salts should be taken to clear any residual allergens out of the bowels.

During the first twenty-four hours, you will experience fairly severe hunger pangs. Although these are quite harmless, they are nevertheless discomforting, so be prepared for them. Drinking water, regularly, will tend to dampen down the desire to eat and, at the same time, cleanse the stomach of irritant juices.

For the person suffering from masked allergies, the second and third days of the fast are the worst. During this time, withdrawal symptoms will be experienced. This is because the food and chemical allergens, in the body, are no longer being masked by ongoing ingestion of these substances. Depending on the range and severity of the illness, symptoms can vary from moderate to extreme, and there is very little one can do, except to rest and ride them out. If the symptoms cause continuing hunger, this can be helped by taking a combination of two parts sodium bicarbonate to one part potassium bicarbonate, in a large glass of pure water. It is advisable to have a chemist make up this formula before starting the fast. Take it as often as you need. It will be of particular help in reducing your cravings for favourite (allergenic) foods, such as bread, chocolate, coffee, etc.

It is important to remember that during the fast all allergenic substances must be avoided. Obviously food will not be eaten, but what about chemicals? The whole purpose of the fast is to clean out toxins and residual allergens from the body. Remember, food sensitivity is invariably accompanied by chemical sensitivity. Therefore, it is necessary to avoid chemical substances as well as food substances. Obviously smoking is out, otherwise tobacco toxins will hamper the cleansing process. By the second or third day, the body will have started to eliminate tobacco residue and chemicals, with which it has been saturated for years. Eventually, the nicotine craving ceases and giving up smoking, permanently, becomes much easier. Remember to drink only purified water, as tap water is likely to be contaminated with chemicals. If you are taking medication, try to avoid doing so for the period of your fast — but check with your doctor first. Medication should also be avoided for the food-testing period if possible.

Other chemicals to be avoided are contained in toothpaste, scented soap, hair tonic, etc. Bad breath will be a problem, however, some assistance can be gained by cleaning the teeth and gargling with sea salt or bicarbonate of soda. Do not take vitamin or mineral supplements. Taking anything but water into your stomach might set off cravings for food, resulting in your body becoming confused and in the cleansing process being interrupted.

Many people suffer withdrawal symptoms during a fast, whether they be burdened with serious allergy illness or not. The reason for this is that nearly all people, who follow modern eating habits, are 'hooked' on one or more food substances without even knowing it. Even a twenty-four hour fast can provoke these symptoms. The 'Yom Kippur headache' is well known in Jews, who fast from one sunset to the following, in observance of this holy day in their religion. Often, it is the first indication the sufferer has that his body has become addicted to a regularly eaten food or favourite drink. Coffee and soft drinks containing caffeine are notable offenders, but it could well be something as seemingly innocent as chicken, tomato sauce or apples. *Prevention* magazine reports on a Californian woman who fasted for *Yom Kippur* and was overcome by sweating and weakness. Laboratory tests showed that she was suffering from insecticide poisoning. As the body drew on her fat reserves for energy, the stored insecticide toxins were released into the blood. It is likely that many people, today, are suffering from this form of toxic overload which causes havoc in the immune system and results in further intolerance to foods and chemicals.

Withdrawal symptoms will usually be similar to the constant, or recurring symptoms, that have plagued you in the past. Up to, and including the third day, the severity will increase, followed by a rapid decline. To feel symptom-free for the first time in years is a marvellous experience. A common symptom is that of headache, which usually occurs during the first twenty-four hours. Migraine sufferers will possibly experience a severe headache during this time, but if they persevere, it should begin to subside after twenty-four hours and finally disappear.

One of the advantages of the fast is weight loss. Many allergic people are prone to puffiness, due to metabolic upset caused by an exhausted immune system. The result is toxin-impregnated fat deposits and an accumulation of 'allergic fluid'. A normal person, with no allergies, would lose, approximately, two and a half kilos over a five-day fast, whilst a very allergic person could lose in excess of ten kilos. A common weight loss is four to six kilos. The resultant feeling of well-being and vitality is truly remarkable.

In extreme cases withdrawal symptoms can be reduced by analgesics. Do not take aspirin, or any pain killer containing salicylates, as these are a well-known allergen. Acupuncture can be extremely useful in minimising withdrawal symptoms, and reference should be made to the chapter on acupuncture. It is not uncommon for feelings of anxiety to be experienced during the first three days of the fast. Persevere with these, because by the fourth or fifth day you should begin to feel much better. If, however the anxiety becomes too much for you, it is far better to ask your doctor for a tranquilliser (such as valium) than to abort the fast. Large doses of vitamin C (10-12 gm per day) and vitamin B complex (200 mg, or more, three times a day) can help reduce withdrawal symptoms if taken three or four consecutive days before the fast begins.

Don't be surprised if you feel cold during your fast. This is usual, and you should keep warm with extra clothing, and should place an extra blanket on the bed. Avoid extremes of temperature. You should not take very hot showers as these will tend to drain your energy, leaving you feeling weak and tired. Above all, consult your doctor, if during the fast you are concerned about your health in any way.

After the fast and reintroduction of foods

At the end of the five-day fast you will be feeling like a completely different person. You will realize that you had forgotten what it was like to feel well. Allergy illness is an insidious business that can overtake you, without your even knowing it. Once free of accumulated allergenic matter, the body and the brain undergo a rebirth. People of all ages experience the transformation to a state of greatly increased mental, and physical, vitality. Food tastes better, digestion is improved, limbs feel lighter, legs stronger and the heartbeat has steadied down to a slower, more even pulse. Handwriting often improves, sometimes dramatically, indicating how the nervous system had become affected by food and chemical allergens in the past.

After the fast, reintroduction of foods is done on the basis of one per day, to allow a full twenty-four hours for allergy symptoms to emerge. Although it means only one food can be eaten on the first day, the second day this food can be eaten with a new food and, on the third day, there will be three foods to eat and so on. It is highly unlikely that allergy reactions will take place during the first few days as only hypo-allergy (low or non-allergy) foods will be introduced at first, so that a basic diet can be built up as soon as possible. If a reaction does take place, then one to three teaspoons of the 2:1 sodium bicarbonate and potassium bicarbonate mixture, in a glass of water, will invariably reduce it.

During the food testing phase, minor set-backs can occur. An encounter with an allergen can leave you feeling cold and exhausted, hot and irritable, sneezing and itching, coughing, tense, nauseous, headachy and many other nasty symptoms. Sometimes, a reaction to one food can set up a craving for quite a different food. Beware of a weakening in resolve! Use the 2:1 mixture to tone down the reaction and flush it through the system quickly with a dose of herbal laxative.

It is important to realize that a period of intense sensitivity will follow a fast and, to a lesser extent, an elimination diet. As a result, reactions to allergenic foods can be quite severe until aborted. However, as the immune system and affected organs gain strength this hypersensitivity begins to dwindle. Therefore, there is no need for alarm or despondency. Hypersensitivity means that your allergies are no longer masked, and you are at the true beginning of the recovery phase.

Unsafe foods should not be reintroduced for a further three months after intitial testing. Careful observation of both pulse rate and symptoms should be made. If still unsafe, wait a further three months and try again. Remember, the longer the period of abstinence from a particular food, the more likely you are to acquire a tolerance to it. It is also important to bear in mind that repeated eating of a previously allergenic food, can reawaken the old allergy.

In the case of masked food allergy, this needs careful watching, as you may be 'hooked' again before you realize it. The safest way to deal with these foods is to eat them irregularly, or on a rotational basis.

If you are unlucky enough to eat an unsafe food unknowingly, then simply stop eating and fast. A one- or two-day fast will be of great assistance in removing the allergens and allowing your system to revert to normality quickly. Take care of your immune system, in this way, and future problems will be minimal.

In order to assist the immune system and the prevention of future toxic overload one should ideally fast for one day each week. Once you are back on a clean diet and no longer manipulated by cravings and withdrawal symptoms this is easy, and is followed by a sense of health and well-being. If you cannot fast weekly, then even one day per fortnight or per month, will be beneficial. Some people may prefer to do a two day fast, once per month, the beneficial effect being similar to four one day fasts. Continued use of fasting, either on a regular basis, or from time to time, will be of immense benefit to sufferers of food and chemical allergies.

Suggested order of food testing

after five-day fast

Day	Food	Day	Food
1	Lamb	16	Beans
2	Potatoes	17	Fish (not shell fish)
3	Lettuce	18	Onions
4	Pears (well washed)	19	Apples (well washed)
5	Cabbage	20	Chicken
6	Beef	21	Rice
7	Carrots	22	Grapes (well washed)
8	Tea or coffee	23	Chocolate
9	Eggs	24	Pork
10	Milk	25	Olive oil (test with a safe food)
11	Peas	26	Tap water
12	Tomatoes	27	Butter
13	Wheat (as a pure wheat cereal)	28	Mushrooms
14	Cane sugar (labelled cane sugar)	29	Nuts
15	Oranges	30	Pineapple

All food must be fresh. Tinned, processed or frozen food is completely unsuitable.

MANAGEMENT
AND TREATMENT

Why not take charge of your body?

> Ninety per cent of all illnesses that people bring to doctors are
> either self limiting or beyond the medical professions' capabilities
> for cure.

This statement from the *New England Journal of Medicine* leads to
the notion that in many cases we will either get better or grow worse
despite medical treatment.

As many of us are wearily aware, most doctors are still unwilling
to accept food allergy as a major cause of illness — probably because
it is not a 'cut-and-dried' situation that can be easily diagnosed and
treated. Often people with genuine food allergies are wrongly told
that they have a psychological problem. It is patently obvious that
conventional medical practitioners have little idea, of understanding,
of food and chemical allergies. They scoff at the idea of environ-
mentally caused illness and their understanding of the
nutritional needs of the human body, fed on a Western diet, is limited.
Professor J.C. Murdoch, of the Otago School of Medicine, commented
on doctors and their attitude to multiple allergy illness: 'People are
being humiliated purely on the grounds, that they have a certain set
of symptoms, which doctors for some reason don't like.' With regard to the inadequacy of conventional medical tests for the problem, he

says: 'If we believe that the patient is wrong and the doctor and the tests are right then we are adrift.' These are comments of a humane and enlightened person — one of the doyens of the medical profession. Surely this is food for thought for all medical practitioners!

Conventional allergy skin tests do not work. Usually, there is only one way to be sure and that is by avoidance of known allergenic foods. When the symptoms have disappeared, commence reintroducing the foods, one at a time. When a food is found to cause symptoms, then you have discovered the culprit. Take care! Often, there may be a number of foods causing similar symptoms. The mere recognition of one may not be enough to solve your problems. Drs Kenyon and Lewith have this to say about allergy illness:

> Our own experience of clinical ecology makes us think twice before ruling out an ecological cause for any symptom complex, and we have been constantly surprised as to how food and/or chemical sensitivities have produced the most bizarre and surprising diseases.

There is such a massive amount of evidence available today, that there can be no longer any doubt that a great number of illnesses (other than those due to injury or genetic defects) stem from toxic overload. Identification and then avoidance, of allergens is the principal method of dealing with this problem.

Once the offending foods have been avoided for a period of up to twelve months, depending on severity, the body will have lost its allergic sensitivity and the food, or foods, can usually be eaten safely. However, it is a mistake to be lulled into a false sense of security. Once you have had a food allergy problem there is always a likelihood that it may reoccur. The best way to prevent this happening is to ensure that the offending foods are not eaten every day. Dr William Philpott says:

> It cannot be over-emphasized that a four-or-more-day rotation of foods (especially symptom-incriminated foods) is of prime importance when attempting to control ecologically the allergic-addictive states. But it would certainly be wrong to conclude that

a rotation diet alone is the cure–all of physical and mental illness. Nutrients in proper amounts and types can help prevent the majority of maladaptive reactions to foods and/or chemicals.

Nutrients and supplements are dealt with at length in Chapter 15. It is important here to look at the most essential management tool for the control of food/chemical allergy, and the maintenance of good health.

The rotation diet

After having successfully recognized which foods are making you ill, the next step is to manage your diet so that the allergic effects can be avoided, particularly, that most insidious and dangerous of things — addiction! After complete avoidance for a period of time, the body loses its sensitivity and can be re-exposed to allergenic foods, on a carefully managed basis. This method is known as the diversified rotation diet.

American allergist, Dr F.L. Leeney, was the first to use this approach and another leading allergist, Dr H. Rinkel, further refined it. He demonstrated that a symptom-producing food does not have to be avoided forever but can be returned to the diet, on a limited basis, after a period of time, during which sensitivity diminishes. He says that foods, giving minor reactions, should be avoided for a minimum of six weeks, and those causing major reactions should be avoided for three months. After that time, the offending foods can be reintroduced into the diet every four days. If reactions occur on this programme, then further avoidance, for another two to three months, is necessary.

The reasoning behind the four-day rotation diet is that it normally takes three days for food to pass through the intestine. As Dr Kenyon says, it may be possible to get away with a three-day rotation, but, as a 'rule of the thumb', four days is safer.

There is always the danger that a person, once allergic to a number of foods, will develop new allergies to other foods, if they are eaten too often. This is because the body deteriorates into an allergenic state, with the immune system becoming overtired and incapable of dealing with the toxic residues found, normally, in safe foods. When an allergy sufferer is forced to give up staple foods, he will often try to compensate by the adoption of new daily staples. For example, he will substitute soy products for milk, beans for grains, chicken for pork and so on. In no time at all his flagging immune system will, again, be overloaded by constant repetition and further allergies will result. The ideal answer to this problem is the four-day or seven-day rotation diet. This method not only rests the immune system, by preventing it being bombarded with the same toxins day after day, but also gives the individual an eating plan which is more interesting, as well as safe.

Drs Kenyon and Lewith list three advantages of the rotation diet:

1 As a diagnostic tool it can unmask hitherto unrecognised, hidden (masked) food allergies.

2 It makes it less likely that the person will develop new allergies to foods which he is regularly in contact with, having substituted these foods in place of allergic foods.

3 It helps the multiple food allergic person to lead a reasonable lifestyle and to maintain tolerance to the food he is already able to eat.

The diversified rotation diet allows the food allergy sufferer to maintain as balanced a nutritional intake as possible. However, sometimes supplements will be needed. Otherwise, as well as developing new allergies, it can be possible to become malnourished very quickly, leading to further aggravation of existing problems.

The principles of rotation diets are as follows:

1 Eat non-processed natural foods — preferably organically grown. Avoid spices, dressings, condiments, etc., as much as possible, but not entirely, as there must be some variety. Avoid composite foods containing several ingredients, such as sausages, packet soups, tinned meats, etc.

2 Vary your diet as much as possible. This can be achieved by looking to other cultures for food ideas. Chinese, Indian and Indonesian cooking contain some varied and harmless foods. These foods may cost a little more, but without health, what is money?

3   The main aim of a rotation diet is to allow your body to recover from the effects of a food, before eating it again. As it takes three days to pass through the intestine, it is important not to eat any food more often than every four days. Otherwise, allergies to previously safe foods can develop. There can be some flexibility to this approach, however, depending on the degree, or severity, of the allergy problem.

4   As well as the food, the food family itself should be rotated. According to Dr Theron Randolph, who is the acknowledged world leader in this field, three main points apply. These are:

I   Any food, whether allergenic or not, should be eaten only once every four days.

II   Foods are established in families, and only one food of any food family from any of these groups should be eaten during a single day.

III   There should be a separation of one day, between any two members of the same food family. For example, wheat could be eaten on the first day and then oats, another member of the cereal-grain family, could be safety eaten on the third day, but not the second day.

If the food family is not rotated in this way, it is likely that sensitivity, to another member of the same family, will quickly develop. For example, potatoes and tomatoes should be eaten a full day apart, as they both belong to the 'potato family'.

5   A rotation diet must, initially, consist only of foods to which you are not allergic. It is usually at least four to six months, before your immune system has recovered to the point where reintroduction of allergenic foods can commence. The important thing is to be flexible. If you find that after a four-day break you get a reaction when you eat the food again, then increase the time delay to seven or eight days. Eventually, you will determine a suitable rotation for that particular food. In most cases, a four-day rotation has proven itself to be adequate for the great majority of food allergies. With extremely sensitive people, who have been sick for a long time, it may be necessary

to use a seven-day rotation. The principle is the same, however, and, eventually, it should be possible to reduce to a four-day rotation, once the immune system has regained some resilience.

Dr Randolph points out that, the smaller the number of foods eaten at any one meal, the less the likelihood of an allergy reaction. However, this usually applies only in severe cases of multiple food allergy.

As we are already aware, allergies may be either 'cyclical', 'transient' or 'fixed'. In the case of the first two, avoidance, followed by a diversified rotation diet will eventually solve the problem. A 'fixed' allergy however, such as some forms of milk intolerance or sensitivity to gluten, is totally incurable. Complete and lifelong avoidance in these cases is the only way to maintain good health. We are fortunate today, to have access to such a wide range of foodstuffs, that even total avoidance of a particular type of food should not prevent us from enjoying our diet and receiving a good level of nourishment. As Dr Kenyon says, the individual's involvement in the treatment of allergy illness, is essential in order to obtain any degree of success. A sensible person should be able to apply the principles of the rotation diet and then work out the rest for himself.

Remember, sensitivity to common staple foods is generally applicable to most people with food allergy problems. Thus, it is a sound idea at first, to avoid them, even if you are not convinced of your allergy to them. An initial rotation diet would be better without wheat, milk, corn, eggs and yeast. Particular care should be taken to avoid these items in composite foods. Subject to your own identified sensitivities, a four-day rotation diet could contain the foods listed on the following page.

This diet is suggested as an example only, and should be varied, according to individual requirements and availability of foodstuffs. (Refer to food families at the end of this chapter.)

It is interesting to note that cooking food in oils, or fats, reduces the absorption rate and this reduces allergic symptoms. Frequent use of oil, however, is not recommended, due to danger of fatty acids, and triglycerides, building up to unhealthy levels in the body.

Four-Day Rotation Diet

Day	Food Family	Food
1	MUSTARD	Broccoli, mustard, cauliflower, turnip
	PALM	Chinese cabbage, radish, horseradish
	PARSLEY	Celery
	FISH	Salmon, perch, bass, other freshwater fish
	MINT	Thyme, marjoram, oregano, peppermint
	CASHEW	Pistachio, mango
	BIRD	Duck, turkey, guinea fowl, goose
	COMPOSITES	Lettuce, sunflower seed, chicory
	PLUM	Nectarine, apricot
	GOURD	Squash, zucchini, rockmelon, honeydew
	MORNING GLORY	Sweet potato
	CITRUS	Grapefruit, citron, lemon, tangerine
	CRUSTACEA	Prawn, shrimp
	OIL	Sunflower
	TEA	Peppermint, dandelion
2	LEGUME	Kidney bean, navy bean, lima bean, lentils, soya bean, blackeyed pea, pea, green bean
	POTATO	Tomato, capsicum, paprika
	GOOSEFOOT	Beetroot, silver beet
	EBONY	Persimmon
	LAUREL	Avacado

	ROSE	Raspberry, blackberry
	APPLE	Apple
	MULBERRY	Fig
	BOVIDAE	Lamb
	SPURGE	Tapioca
	LILY	Leek, garlic
	SUIDAE	Pork
	OIL	Soybean, lamb fat
	TEA	Alfalfa
3	PLUM	Cherry, peach, plum, almond, apricot
	BIRD	Chicken, pheasant, quail
	CITRUS	Orange, lime
	PAWPAW	Pawpaw
	COMPOSITES	Artichoke, endive, safflower
	CRUSTACEA	Crayfish, crab
	MUSTARD	Lettuce, cabbage, Brussels sprouts, watercress
	PALM	Coconut, date
	GOURD	Pumpkin, cucumber, watermelon, squash
	PARSLEY	Carrot, parsley, parsnip, dill, coriander, cumin
	FISH	Whiting, cod, herring, tuna, other saltwater fish
	MINT	Basil, sage, spearmint
	OLIVE	Olives (black and green)
	OIL	Olive, coconut
	TEA	Spearmint
4	BUCKWHEAT	Rhubarb, buckwheat
	LEGUME	Peanut
	POTATO	Potato, eggfruit
	GOOSEFOOT	Spinach
	LILY	Asparagus, onion, chive
	MULBERRY	Mulberry, breadfruit
	BOVIDAE	Beef, butter, cheese

APPLE	Pear
MOLLUSC	Mussel, oyster, squid, snail, abalone, scallop
BANANA	Banana
ROSE	Strawberry, boysenberry
GRAPE	Grapes, raisins, sultanas
CEREAL	Rice, millet, bamboo shoots
OIL	Peanut, beef fat
TEA	Strawberry leaf, rosehip

It is not necessary to eat from all the food families indicated, each day.

About once a fortnight if things are going well on the diet, you should have a break from it and go out to dinner. Everyone needs a reward now and again. Obviously, you should not eat anything to which you are severely allergic, but after a few months on the four-day rotation diet, you should build up enough resistance to break it occasionally. As a safeguard against allergic reactions on these occasions, it is a good idea to fortify oneself, before, during and after the meal, with appropriate nutrients. Various researchers have found, that, several grams of Vitamin C, plus pancreatic enzymes, taken one hour before the meal, together with further pancreatic enzymes and bicarbonate of soda taken about half an hour after the meal, can have an anti-allergy effect. It is also a good idea, to take vitamin B Complex during the meal.

Very sensitive people can safeguard themselves further against an allergy reaction by taking an anti-inflammatory agent such as Heparin. About 2500 units would be appropriate. In much higher doses, Heparin is used as an anti-coagulant, and for this reason it can only be obtained by medical prescription.

Another anti-inflammatory agent of equal value, in reducing reactions to foods and chemicals, is Procaine, which has been used for years, and with some success, in Rumania and other European countries, to retard the ageing process.

Desensitisation

This process can be carried out by clinical ecologists who are trained medical doctors, specialising in a far more sophisticated approach to food and chemical allergies, than hitherto followed by conventional medicine. Unfortunately, there are too few of these, much needed people presently practising outside Britain and America. The procedure basically involves desensitisation, using sublingual drops made up from samples of the allergen. Various testing methods, including autonomic cardiac response and VEGATEST EAV equipment can assess the 'end point' — which is, basically, the strength of solution needed to commence the desensitisation process. The drops are taken three times per day, over a period of time, during which the patient is retested, several times, and the strength of the drops is progressively increased.

Some people have had their food allergies removed in this manner, but, because of the diversity of causes of allergy illness, not all people can be helped in this way. The procedure is generally more successful with chemical allergies, and can even be used for inhaled sensitivities, such as exhaust fumes and tobacco smoke.

Hair analysis

This analysis is an extremely useful method of assessing mineral balance in the body, as well as monitoring levels of toxic metals, such as lead and mercury. It involves burning a sample of hair and analysing the ash, using spectro-photometry.

The importance of this procedure, to multiple allergy sufferers, cannot be over-emphasised. Clinical ecologists have found that attention to underlying deficiencies and toxicities pays big dividends in health improvement and in resurgence of vitality in the immune system.

Mineral deficiency and toxicity in people is very common. It is a classic example of how our modern food sources cannot supply the body adequately with the proper mineral nutrients it needs. Remember, the body is basically a chemical factory. Without the right ingredients, it simply cannot produce the necessary chemical reactions for proper operation.

Some examples of mineral toxicity that can be ascertained by hair analysis are:

Arsenic & Mercury — Which come from a wide range of industrial sources as well as tinned tuna and other foodstuffs. Raised levels of these metals in the blood, contribute to toxic overload with all its attendant problems. This is a common situation.

Lead — Raised lead levels are also a very common problem — extremely harmful to the nervous system and has a depressant effect on the immune system.

Copper — Raised copper levels are not uncommon and are associated with the contraceptive pill, intra-uterine devices, copper water pipes, etc. Usually, when copper is raised, that most important of minerals, zinc, is either low or not being used properly. Vitamin C supplements assist the body to absorb more copper.

Examples of mineral deficiency are:

Chromium — A lowered level of this mineral indicates a problem with the handling of carbohydrates. As we have seen carbohydrate intolerance is a major cause of food allergy. Many people have this problem without knowing it.

Manganese — Less than normal levels of this mineral have been associated with reduction in short term memory and 'cracking joints'. Manganese deficiency is so widespread that Dr P.J. Kingsley, a noted clinical ecologist in Britain, reports that: 'It is very rare indeed to see a normal manganese level and the reason seems to be that processed food is very low in manganese.'

Dr Kingsley goes on to say that manganese supplementation in autistic children produced clinical improvement. Today there is an indisputable mass of evidence to show that autism, and other bizarre behaviour in both children and adults, is caused by food intolerance and the resultant malabsorption of nutrients.

Zinc — This mineral is essential for about 150 different enzyme processes in the body. For various reasons, hair analysis is not particularly accurate in identifying zinc deficiency. Suffice to say, however, that most modern diets contain less than a minimum daily requirement. Bearing in mind that damage to the gut and malabsorption, caused by ecological illness, result in deficiencies anyway, a daily supplement of zinc should be taken as a matter of course. Zinc is one of the most important minerals in the human body and an adequate supply is absolutely vital to ensure efficient functioning of the immune system.

Selenium — This is a very important and, sometimes under-rated, mineral. It is important in the maintenance of correct pancreatic function, which is absolutely vital in the treatment of allergy illness. Cancer conditions always show low selenium levels. Supplementation should be in conjunction with daily doses of vitamin E.

These are some examples of the usefulness of hair analysis. Assessment of mineral levels, and toxicity, is a valuable guide to whether the body is working efficiently or not. Low levels of minerals clearly indicate malabsorption and food/chemical intolerance. High levels of toxic metals indicate malfunction of the immune system and a body which is biochemically out of balance.

The procedure for taking a hair sample is simple. The hair should be about 2.5cm long and cut as close to the scalp as possible. The best place to take a sample is along the nape of the neck. Hair analysis can be carried out every six months. Because of anomalies, which can only be interpreted correctly by an orthomolecular physician, or a clinical ecologist, it is pointless to consult your average general practitioner on this matter.

The major tool for the management of food allergies is the four-day, or seven-day, rotation diet. Chemical allergies, on the other hand, may often be treated by various forms of desensitization. Other techniques are now being evolved by clinical ecologists to assist in the management and treatment of allergy illness. These techniques are in new fields of medicine which are destined to leave the ineffective, dangerous, drug-oriented approach of today, far behind.

Food Families

APPLE	Apple: cider, pectin, vinegar — pear, quince (also seeds)
ARROWROOT	Dasheen — poi — taro root
BANANA	Banana — plantain
BIRCH	Hazelnuts
BRAZIL NUT	Brazil nut
BUCKWHEAT	Buckwheat — garden sorrel — rhubarb
CACTUS	Prickly pear — tequila
CAPER	Caper
CAROB	Carob
CASHEW	Cashew — mango — pistachio
CEREAL	Bamboo shoots — barley: malt — cane: molasses, sugar — corn: cerelose, cornmeal, corn oil, cornstarch, corn syrup, dextrose, glucose.
	Millett — oats — rice — rye — sorghum.
	Wheat: bran, farina, flour and gluten, wheatgerm.
	Wild rice
CHICORY	Chicory
CITRUS	Angostura bitters — citrange — citron — grapefruit — kumquat — lemon — lime — mandarin — orange — tangerine
COCHLIOSPERNUM	Gum guaiac — gum karaya
COMPOSITE FAMILY	Absinthe — artichoke — celtuse — chamomile — chickory — dandelion — endive — escarole — goldenrod — head lettuce — jerusalem artichoke — leaf lettuce — oyster plant — safflower oil — sesame seeds: hummus, oil, tahini — sunflower seeds: oil — tarragon — vermouth:

	cragweed, pyrethrum
EBONY	Persimmon
FUNGUS	Mushroom — yeast
GINGER	Cardomom — ginger — tumeric
GOOSEBERRY	Currant — gooseberry
GOOSEFOOT (Beet)	Beetroot: sugar — chard — kochia — lamb's quarters — Silver beet — spinach — thistle
GOURD	Cantaloupe — casaba melon — cucumber — honey-dew melon — muskmelon — Persian melon — pumpkin — squash — watermelon
GRAPE	Brandy — cream of tartar — grapes — raisins — sultanas — wine: champagne — wine vinegar
HEATH	Blueberry — cranberry — huckleberry — wintergreen
HOLLY	Bearberry — mate — pokeberry
HONEYSUCKLE	Elderberry
IRIS	Saffron
LAUREL	Avocado — bay leaves — cassia bark — cinnamon — sassafras
LEGUME	Black-eyed peas — carob — chick peas — field peas — green peas — gum acacia — gum tragacanth — kidney beans — lentil — licorice — lima beans — mung beans — navy beans — peanuts: oil, paste — pinto beans — snow peas — soy beans: flour, lecithin, oil — string beans — tamarind
LILY	Asparagus — chives — garlic — leek — onion — sarsaparilla — shallots
MADDER	Coffee
MALLOW	Cottonseed — maple syrup: sugar — okra
MAY APPLE	May apple herb
MINT	Basil — oregano — horehound —

	majoram — peppermint — sage — savory — thyme
MORNING GLORY	Sweet potato
MULBERRY	Breadfruit — fig — hop — mulberry
MUSTARD	Broccoli — brussels sprouts — cabbage — cauliflower — kale — mustard — mustard greens — rutabagas (swede turnips) — turnips
MYRTLE	Allspice — cloves — guava: cherry guava
NUTMEG	Mace — nutmeg
OAK	Chestnuts
OLIVE	Green, black, olive oil
ORCHID	Vanilla
PALM	Celery cabbage — chinese cabbage — coconut — collard — colza shoots — date — horseradish — kohlrabi — kraut — palm cabbage — radish — sago — watercress
PARSLEY	Angelica — anise — caraway — carrots — celeriac — celery — celery seed — coriander — cumin — dill — fennel — parsley — parsnips — water celery
PAWPAW	Papain — papaya — pawpaw
PEPPER	Black and white and green
PINE	Juniper berry (gin) — pinion nut: pignolia
PINEAPPLE	Pineapple
PLUM	Almond — apricot — cherry — nectarine — peach — persimmon — plum: prune — wild cherry
POMEGRANATE	Pomegranate
POPPYSEED	Poppyseed
POTATO	Belladonna — chilli — eggplant — green pepper — ground cherry — hyoscyamus — potato — red pepper: capsicum, cayenne — starmonium

	(datura) — tobacco — tomato
PURSLANE	New Zealand spinach — purslane
ROSE	Blackberry — boysenberry — dewberry — loganberry — raspberry — strawberry — youngberry
SAPODILLA	Chicle
SOAPBERRY	Lychee nuts
STERCULA	Cocoa: chocolate — cola bean
SPURGE	Kassava meal — tapioca
TEA	Tea
WALNUT	Black walnut — butternut — English walnut — hickory — pecan

14

CORRECT EATING AND NUTRITION

Some startling facts

Much has been said in earlier chapters, about the need to eat correctly — that is, not only to refrain from eating chemical-laden junk, but also, to take careful note that some of the, so-called 'good foods' can be just as harmful to some people as chemical-containing processed foods.

Chemical additives silt up the cells and prevent the body's biochemistry from functioning efficiently. Toxic overload results, we get sick and stay sick, even though we may still be holding down a job. How many people arrive home from work, tired, irritable and really unable to enjoy the remainder of their day? They will go through the motions of having a good time because it is expected of them, when, often, they would prefer to slump in front of the TV or go to bed. There are a great many people with this problem, unaware that their bodies are overloaded by toxic junk, due to wrong eating. They do not understand that what is good for someone else may not be good for them. It is a fact that some people may get away with the most atrocious diets for, perhaps, most of their life. However, most of us, if we are to lead a long and robust life, free from toxic overload and allergy illness must take careful note of our individual, nutritional needs and limitations.

For many people, a so-called normal diet, will produce reactions and side effects simply because they have, unknowingly, become intolerant, or allergic, to some of their daily foods.

Dr M.B. Cambell writes, in *Allergy of the Nervous System*, that observation has shown that 69 per cent of all headaches are ecologically caused, (i.e. nutrition, environment, etc). However, Dr William Philpott, a leading allergist in the United States, says, on headaches, that the chance of the average general practitioner or specialist looking to nutrition and environment for the cause, is slim. The majority of doctors still persist in looking for a specific disease-linked cause, and the victim ends up being palliated with drugs. A recent research programme, carried out at the National Hospital for Nervous Diseases, in London, proved that headaches are commonly caused by food allergies. It found that the offending foods could be colourings, food additives, sugar, tea, coffee, alcohol, milk and milk products, grains and cereals, meats, fruit pips and nuts. All foods commonly found in our everyday diet.

According to researchers at Sydney Hospital, one-third of Australians are addicted to caffeine. These people drink a minimum of five cups of tea, or coffee, per day. They have shown that the side effects suffered, contribute to degenerative disease and allergy illness. In other words, one of the most common items in our daily diet can be the cause of illness for a third of the population.

The four basic foods fallacy

The conventional medical approach on diet and nutrition, is that we should eat something from each of the four basic foods every day. These, so-called, four basic foods are:

1 Grains and cereals
2 Milk and dairy products
3 Meat, fish and poultry
4 Fruit and vegetables

During the course of our schooling, it was emphasised that unless we ate of the four basic foods each day, we could not hope to keep healthy. In adulthood, we find that the brainwashing continues with advertising, articles and propaganda from health organisations, all aimed at perpetuating the myth of the four-foods basis for a wholesome diet. As a consequence, a great majority of people are totally encapsulated by this philosophy. The tragedy, of course, is that many people are allergic to at least two of these four foods, namely, milk and dairy products, and grains and cereals.

Today, our whole social structure revolves around the 'four-foods philosophy'. So much so, that were this to be changed overnight, our national, social and economic infrastructure would collapse and total chaos would result. Why? Because a substantial part of our free enterprise economy, throughout both primary and secondary industry, is involved in the production and processing of vast amounts of each of the four foods. 'Feed the man meat!' 'Milk is good for you!' 'Bread is the staff of life!' These messages, in various forms, are presented to us dozens of times each day, absolutely entrenching, our belief that the foods they represent are essential to our well-being. What chance then, does the average person have to consider seriously, that he or she may be allergic to the very foods that are, literally, the basis of our whole way of life? The possibility that one, two or even three, of the basic four foods could be dispensed with, and yet good health be maintained, is a concept so fantastic as to be totally unacceptable to most people.

Ross Horne, in *The New Health Revolution*, has cited numerous, well researched and authoritative sources to show that meat, grain and dairy products can be the cause of a wide range of degenerative diseases, due to the body developing intolerances and, as a result, becoming overloaded with toxins. This does not necessarily mean that these foods should never be eaten, but indicates that caution should be applied. The heavy emphasis on meat, dairy products and refined grains, in Australia and other countries, has been shown to be a major cause of degenerative disease — and of course, this starts by the body becoming first sensitive and then allergic to the offending food.

As we have seen in the past chapters, intolerance and allergy to foods comes about because of the body's inability to process certain foods properly. This can be due to a variety of reasons. The result is that undigested food particles enter the bloodstream and wreak havoc throughout the body. These toxins continue to accumulate in the body, lowering tolerance, wrecking the immune system and finally evolving into specific disease which can result in death. This whole process can take many, many years, during which time the quality of life is gradually destroyed. For some, this can happen much earlier than for others, and it is all directly linked with diet.

Correct eating and nutrition must be entirely an individual approach. However, there are known guidelines which should be examined by people who feel that their bodies are not giving them the health and energy that is rightfully theirs. For a start, the whole idea of the 'four-foods' basis for health and nutrition needs careful examination. The following points show why:

Grains and cereals Reference has been made in earlier chapters, to the fact that grains and cereals are a proven allergen and one of the most common known to man. Furthermore, it is possible to be addicted to grains without realizing it. Addiction is linked directly with allergy, as one always exists with the other. Adverse reactions to grains can be extremely subtle, and it is often very difficult for individuals to link grain allergy with specific health problems. Grain allergies can vary from slight to severe. Symptoms can range from overweight, tiredness, mental illness, to chronic disease. There is one thing that is certain in our grain-eating oriented society and that is — **We eat too much grain and cereal and this is causing health problems for a great many people.**

Some people are allergic to all grains, others to specific grains. The worst common offender is wheat. Dr Philpott in his book, *Brain Allergies*, feels that wheat causes more problems than any other allergenic substance. He says, 'In my studies, wheat is seen to be the highest maladaptive reacting substance, especially in invoking mental symptoms.'

Writing in his book, *Health for Life*, Dr William Vayda refers to the wheat problem as, 'A disorder being increasingly diagnosed in the Western world, due to the vastly increased consumption of wheat products, beyond the levels the human body was designed to handle.'

Although cereals provide the bulk of diet for many people world wide, it cannot be said to be a natural food for humans. In terms of human evolution, it is only a 'moment' since man began to cultivate and eat grains, prodigiously. Prior to a few thousand years ago, he subsisted, for six million years, on hunting and gathering. During this time, cereals played only a very minor part in his daily diet. Therefore, in terms of evolution, the human body has not yet had time to develop mechanisms to handle properly, the copious quantities of cereal and grain products that are eaten today.

With the exception of millet and buckwheat (not a true grain), grains are acid-forming in the body. Even when cooked, they are, comparatively, difficult to digest and can produce abdominal swelling and flatulence. Because they are a seed, they contain an enzyme inhibitor, which is not easily broken down, even by cooking. This places a great strain on the pancreas and liver, resulting in a build-up of toxins in the body. Studies, made by various medical researchers, have shown that cereals, wheat in particular, cause deposits of calcium salts in the tissues, leading to degeneration and hardening of the arteries.

Reference was made, in an earlier chapter, to Dr Edward Howell, of Florida, in the United States. In his book, *The Status of Food Enzymes in Digestion and Metabolism*, he referred to research done on the Malays and Filipinos. These people subsisted mainly on rice, and it was found that they eventually developed marked hypertrophy (enlargement) of the pancreas. When this occurs, it indicates that the pancreas is overworked and, in the case of these people, it was due to the huge volume of enzymes that their pancreases had to produce, in order to digest their rice intake. It was found that, whilst Malays and Filipinos had about 50 per cent enlargement, the average American, also, had an enlarged pancreas. When you consider the enormous exposure in our Western diet to processed foods, which contain cereals as fillers, plus the average daily intake of breakfast cereals, bread, biscuits, cakes, etc, it would be surprising if our own intake of cereals is very much less than that of subsistence rice eaters.

People who have a, largely, grain-based diet do not live long lives. They tend to be active up to middle age, but after that, deteriorate quickly. The excessive strain, placed on the human body by a substantial daily intake of cereal and grain products, eventually wears it out. It has been found that an enlarged pancreas will steadily deteriorate in function after middle age, unless it is relieved of the continuous overload placed on it by daily grain consumption.

Wheat, in particular, is a renowned allergen. It has been estimated that 30 per cent of all people are allergic to wheat in some way. The degree of allergy varies, considerably, between individuals. Some should never eat it. Others may eat it fairly regularly but not every day. Grains in general, and wheat in particular, should be eaten sparingly, and certainly not every day, if the body is to cope satisfactorily with them. Otherwise intolerance and allergy may develop, resulting in a progressive and subtle deterioration in health.

A common fallacy is that cereals and grains are necessary to provide enough carbohydrate and fibre. This is not so. An adequate supply of fibre and carbohydrate, can be obtained by substituting fresh fruit and vegetables. An added advantage is that, in their raw state, they are easily digestible, due to the enzymes they contain, thus aiding the pancreas and enhancing nutrient absorption and good health.

However, if you feel that you can tolerate cereal and grain products (preferably not daily), then you should eat wholemeal and whole flour products which have greater nutritional and fibre content. White flour is virtually useless as a food. It is really just a 'filler', and places a great burden on the whole digestive system. Some people with grain allergies can react far less severely to refined white flour, than to wholemeal flour. This should not be taken as a reason for eating white flour regularly. Its nutritional value is so low, that it is pointless to eat it often, and to do so can be detrimental to good health.

Dr David Reuben, whose books have sold over 6 million copies, has this to say about white flour in his book, *Everything You Always Wanted to Know About Nutrition*:

Flour millers like to store flour for long periods of time so they can buy it cheap and sell it at high prices . . . so they remove the wheat germ and bran, leaving only the next to worthless pale, white, starchy endosperm. Endosperm keeps almost forever. Why does endosperm keep so well? Because bugs don't eat it. Because there isn't enough nutrition in a ton of white flour to keep one teenie weenie bug alive. A diet of so-called bread made from white flour — taken right off the supermarket shelves — can't keep laboratory animals alive and it can't keep your children alive.

On the process of 'enrichment' of white flour, he found that,

In the process of milling, over twenty-six essential elements are totally or partially removed from the flour. The laughable process of 'enrichment' puts back about one-sixth of a cents worth of cheap, synthetic vitamins consisting of thiamine, riboflavin and niacin. They also dump in little tiny bits of iron, often in the form of iron filings. If someone pulled twenty-six of your teeth and gave you four little false teeth in return, would you consider your mouth to have been 'enriched'?

This questionable process of 'enrichment' also applies to breakfast cereal,

> There is no category of food product on the market that is more expensive, more profitable and more nutritionally disastrous, than breakfast cereals.

> Breakfast 'cereal' is a fascinating product: refined sugar and refined flour mixed with hydrogenated oil and salt. It contains more artificial colouring than vitamins, is almost 90 per cent starch and sugar and is preserved with chemicals that poison test animals.

Milk and dairy products For a variety of reasons, explained in Chapter 8 and elsewhere, milk is a potent allergen to some people. Cow's milk, fed too early to unsuspecting infants, can damage their digestive systems and render them either allergic, or sensitive, to milk for life. Dr Reuben says:

> Cow's milk — from the dairy and in baby formulas — is one of the primary causes of allergies in babies . . . Human babies fed on breast milk have almost 100 per cent freedom from intestinal infections, far fewer respiratory infections and almost total immunity to allergies.

Pasteurized milk is difficult to digest, even for people who are tolerant to it, due to the fact that the pasteurization process destroys the thirty-five natural enzymes which are found in all raw milk. The most important of these is lipase which breaks down fat and, thus prevents undigested fat globules entering the bloodstream and overstressing the immune system, causing dangerously high levels of cholesterol to accumulate. These enzymes are needed by the body to digest milk, by breaking it down into lactose and other components. Without them, the digestive organs are forced to work harder than they were meant to, causing them to be overstressed and contributing to dysfunction in later life.

In a medical paper, 'The Effect of Heat Processed Foods and Metabolized Vitamin D Milk, on the Dentofacial Structures of Experimental Animals', Dr Francis Pottenger described tests on cats where one group was fed only raw milk and others, pasteurized and processed milks. All generations on the raw milk thrived. The others, however, progressively deteriorated and developed severe defects and disease, over two generations. The third generation (of which only a few survived), was so afflicted that there was no attempt, by the survivors, to produce a fourth generation.

An example of milk allergy causing mental illness, is described in a paper by Dr Maurice Bowerman, of Beaverton, Oregon. He referred to five of his psychiatric patients who for years had suffered from confusion, detachment, poor memory, poor mental efficiency and paranoia. When milk was removed from their diets, four completely recovered, and the other improved significantly. I wonder how many unfortunate people, throughout the world, are being wrongly diagnosed and treated, by psychiatrists, who are not aware of the devastating effects of food and chemical allergies?

Dr William Philpott points out that milk allergies and grain allergies, often go hand in hand. This is due to the damage done to the upper intestinal tract by allergic reactions to grain. The intestine loses its ability to produce the, all-essential, lactase enzyme, plus many others that are necessary to digest milk. Thus, milk becomes a poison with devastating effects on both physical and mental health.

It is a fallacy that people outgrow milk sensitivity. If you had trouble with milk as a child, then you will have trouble as an adult. The tragedy of it is that many people, as children, were milk-allergic, but that fact was never realized by doctor or parents. Now, as adults, they continue to deteriorate and are usually addicted, without knowing it, to a wide range of dairy products, such as cheese, ice cream, puddings and virtually anything with milk in it.

Another cause of milk allergy is galactosemia which occurs, sometimes hereditarily, when the liver is unable to change galactose into glucose. All dairy products, except cheddar cheese, contain galactose, although the amount of galactose in butter is negligible; so that people with this problem, can usually eat some cheddar cheese and butter, if they scrupulously avoid all other dairy products.

The important thing to remember is that milk is the second major allergenic food. Reactions to it are often not obvious, and there is a wide range, in the degree of allergy, from slight through to severe. Even the most severe allergy may be in the form of a masked addiction so that, neither the sufferer, nor his conventional medical practitioner can relate the problem to his chronic and, perhaps, bizarre physical and mental condition. As Dr Reuben says, 'Adults do not need milk.' Nevertheless, milk and milk products are very attractive foods and may be eaten by some people without harm.

It is a mistake, however, to eat dairy products on a daily basis. Like cereals, they should be eaten sparingly and if possible, only raw milk and raw milk products should be taken. If you have any suspicion at all of food-related health problems, you should treat all milk and dairy products as prime suspects until proven otherwise.

The old pedantism, that dairy products are essential for the maintenance of good health, is a fallacy, perpetrated by bureaucrats and medical people, who find it easier to mouth the same old, outdated health platitudes than to bother taking note of progress in the real world of scientific knowledge. To quote Dr Walter Alvarez, a leading American psychiatrist and allergist: 'We doctors are the most stubborn lot in the world! Many doctors are so stubborn as to think that a fact can't be true if they were not taught it in medical school.'

For example, the main argument in the past has been that milk is an essential source of calcium and phosphorous. For a start, modern scientific research has shown that we need a lot less calcium than was originally thought. In fact, too much calcium is dangerous, because it can damage the kidneys and cause kidney stones, which can virtually ruin your life. Calcium is stored well by the body, so you don't have to eat it every day. What most people do not realize is that an average daily diet, without milk, contains far more calcium than the body can use. In fact, your body rejects about 80 per cent of all calcium you eat, in order to keep your blood concentration relatively low. Such foods as whole wheat bread, beans, olives, peanuts and dozens of other vegetables, contain more calcium than the average person can use.

The same applies to phosphorous. It is almost impossible to become deficient in phosphorous, and an adequate diet of fruit and vegetables will provide ample quantities for good health. It is the belief of Dr Reuben that 'Everybody doesn't need milk and more than half the people in the world — including nearly a quarter of the people in the United States — can get sick if they drink milk.'

Meat, fish and poultry To quote Lady Phyllis Cilento, in reply to a question on whether she ate meat: 'What's wrong with a good steak?' Obviously, nothing is wrong with a good steak, as Lady Cilento, a medical doctor is ninety-one and still puts in a good day's work. She admits, however, that she eats meat sparingly, takes daily nutrient supplements and eats plenty of fresh fruit and vegetables. Her attitude towards meat is, undoubtedly, the correct one. There is just too much evidence, today, against a high meat diet being good for you. A lot of meat in the diet is particularly bad for allergy sufferers because it places a greater strain on bodily functions, already overstressed by constant allergic reactions. For example:

— Too much meat can cause inflammation of the nervous system.

— Aggravation of myxoedema is caused by a diet relatively high in meat. (Myxoedema is linked to thyroid dysfunction and metabolism disorders.)

— Vital organs are overstressed by a high level of toxins from meat. (Remember, toxic overload and allergy illness are partners).

— A high meat diet can cause gout and arteriosclerosis.

— A high meat diet can cause cancer.

— Diabetes, which is strongly linked to food allergy illness, can be both aggravated and caused, by a high meat diet.

— The blood is thickened and circulation reduced. (This also happens to food allergy sufferers due to undigested, or waste matter remaining in their blood.)

— Meat produces acids which are destructive, unless counteracted by adequate fresh fruit and vegetables.

— Meat does not stimulate bowel movement, and transit through the body is slow.

— Accumulated toxins from the slow bowel process, are reabsorbed into the body, placing a great strain on liver and kidneys.

— The thyroid gland, liver and pancreas become damaged, and altered, on a high meat diet.

It is easy to see, therefore, why too much meat should be viewed with caution. In addition to the natural toxins accumulated in the body, due to excessive meat consumption, there is the added danger of the chemicals associated with modern-day meat production. Meat tends to be loaded with dangerous chemicals, such as the carcinogen diethylstilbestrol, residues of DDT and other pesticides, as well as all the antibiotics that are pumped into animals these days to reduce mortality rates during growth.

A further factor adding to toxic overload, is that of sodium nitrite and sodium nitrate, which are, invariably, added to processed meats such as ham, bacon and sausages. Experiments at Michael Reese Hospital, in Chicago, have shown that these chemicals form cancer-producing compounds, in the body, which an overloaded immune system may not have the ability to throw out. Research carried out at the New York State College of Agriculture and Life Sciences, concluded that food additives and high protein diets were the main causes of cancer. Cornell University scientist, Dr T.C. Cambell, agrees; he says that low meat diets, combined with plenty of fresh fruit and vegetables, prevented toxic overload in the body. He also recommended supplements of vitamins A, C and E.

There is no doubt that meat is an excellent source of protein, and there is no reason why it should not continue to provide protein in a healthy, allergy-free diet, but not every day ! Australians, on the average, consume about 100 grams of protein per day. This is three to four times more than the average daily requirement. The Pritikin Foundation says, diets containing more than 20 per cent protein (from all sources), cause a loss of essential minerals. Dr Sheldon Margen, Professor of Nutrition at the University of California, follows this theory. Dr Margen thinks that a 10 per cent protein intake is better. He makes the point that babies have no trouble growing on mothers' milk which contains only 6 per cent protein. People become supremely healthy on the Pritikin diet, with an intake of only 120 grams of lean meat per week!

It is suspected that a high protein diet is destructive to the body. Amongst other things, too much protein causes acidity and the passage of extra calcium through the kidneys, via the urine. Kidney stones, together with reduced kidney function, can result.

It is interesting to note that Eskimos traditionally live on a diet which is extremely high in meat. The difference is, however, that the majority of their meat is consumed raw. Whereas cooked meat contains no enzymes, raw meat contains the proteolytic enzyme, cathepsin and the fat-digesting enzyme, adipose lipase. These enzymes play a major part in digestion in the stomach. Thus, when the meat reaches the intestine, digestion is completed much more efficiently, resulting in less toxic residue. Even so, Eskimos do not lead long lives. To quote one researcher: 'Old age sets in at fifty and its signs are strongly marked at sixty. Comparatively few live beyond sixty and only a very few reach seventy. People who lead vigorous outdoor lives, are usually healthy in old age, if their diet is sound.' One of the best examples of this is the Hunzas, a small nation of people who live in the Himalaya Mountains. (See Chapter 19, on Exercise). It seems valid to suspect, therefore, that the almost total reliance on meast by Eskimos, could have something to do, with the relative shortness of their lifespan.

Animal proteins can cause toxic overload and be destructive to good health, if eaten to excess. They are best eaten sparingly, and certainly not every day. It is possible to keep in superb health without any animal protein at all. The body requires comparatively small amounts of protein to stay healthy and this can be easily derived from a diet of fresh fruits and vegetables, some grains, or as an alternative, beans, little or no dairy produce and very little meat.

Fish and poultry should always be considered as alternatives to red meat. The sad fact about poultry is that, in our chemically mad world, it is usually loaded with antibiotics, hormones and the residues of feed, containing arsenic and a host of other chemicals. Free-range chickens are much safer. Fish, on the other hand, is relatively free from such chemicals and toxins. However in some parts of the world, they have a dangerously high mercury content, due to industrial effluent contaminating their natural habitat.

Some people may react to certain natural chemicals in fish, which can produce numbness, itchiness, joint and muscle pains, fatigue, diarrhoea, nausea, headache and chills. According to Dr Noel Gillespie, of the University of Queensland, the safest way to eat fish is:

1 Not every day
2 Not too much at one meal
3 Not the same variety each time.

Fruit and vegetables In recent years it has been shown, time and time again by researchers, that the ultimate diet for the onward maintenance of good health, is one that consists mainly of fresh fruit and vegetables. Possibly Dr Gerson and Nathan Pritikin have led the way, in this respect, with their remarkable successes with cancer and heart attack patients.

In earlier chapters, the subject of toxic overload, due to allergic reactions from wrong diet and chemicals, was dealt with at some length. Furthermore, Dr Mackarness' 'water in the barrel' principle indicated that, if enough allergens, and food/chemical intolerances, could be recognized and removed, from an individual's diet, then his immune system would regain enough strength to deal with the remainder. By far the least toxic, and the most nutritional of the four basic foods are fruit and vegetables. While it would bore many people, it is substantiated, scientific fact that a diet of only fruit and vegetables, eaten mainly raw, is by far the healthiest diet that any human being can possibly have. It is possible, however, to achieve excellent allergy-free health simply by cutting right back on the other three basic foods and using fruit and vegetables as the bulk of your diet. Periodic introduction of the others, on a weekly basis, as opposed to a daily basis, can then provide the variety that people, brought up in the Western world, usually crave.

Fruit and vegetables also contain substances that can cause allergy illness. However, if the body is free from toxic assault, from other food/chemical sources, it can usually cope. An example of such substances is the salicylates found in apples, apricots, berries, cherries, grapes, nectarines, peaches and plums. My own experiences have shown that the 'Mackarness theory' holds true. At my worst, I found that these fruits caused me a variety of discomforting reactions, such as headache, drowsiness and irritability, often with a lingering aftermath. These symptoms are uncomfortable, but often subtle, and if you are not 'switched on' to food allergy you tend to dismiss the sensation as just feeling a bit 'off colour'. The underlying problem continues and, gradually worsens over the years. However, once I became aware of the whole food/chemical allergy problem, I began dispensing with the more obvious allergens, such as grains, dairy products, chemicals, processed foods, etc. As my immune system gradually recovered, I noticed an improvement in my tolerance to salicylate-containing fruits. Today, even though I must continue to avoid grain and dairy products (with the occasional exception) I find I can now eat all these fruits with impunity, providing I don't eat them to excess. The point I wish to make here is that, generally speaking, the human body can overcome intolerance to fruit and vegetable toxins, once it is relieved of the more potent toxins, from other foods.

For food/chemical allergy sufferers, a largely vegetarian diet is often the best answer, perhaps supplemented, if tolerance allows, by a small, irregular quantity of the other basic foods. Beware! Do not confuse grain and cereal products with fruit and vegetables. They should always be viewed as a separate food category, and eaten only to the degree that your tolerance of them will allow. Dr Philpott says:

> Classical vegetarians are heavy users of cereal grains and often rely on wheat gluten as a basic source of protein; this leaves the vegetarian who may be genetically programmed as a reactor to wheat in a vulnerable position, since he is more prone to use wheat and other gluten-bearing cereal grains.

Recent studies reported in the *Journal of the American Medical Association*, *The American Journal of Clinical Nutrition*, the *British Journal of Human Nutrition* and the *New England Journal of Medicine* have shown that vegetarians:

1 Are much less affected by allergies
2 Have cleaner blood and lower blood pressure
3 Are slimmer in every age group
4 Have lower cholesterol in their blood, and
5 Are less likely to die of heart attacks.

In addition, women have less oestregen in their blood, and lower incidence of breast cancer. Other studies have shown that vegetarians, who minimise their intakes of grain and dairy products, are the healthiest people of all.

Another study in the United States, recently showed that only 2 per cent of vegetarians had hypertension, as compared with 26 per cent, in the non-vegetarian group. For allergy sufferers, this is significant. Hypertension is one of the classic symptoms of ecological illness. Researchers from Addenbrooke's Hospital, in Cambridge, have linked low incidence of strokes to a predominance of fresh fruit and vegetables in the diet. This is because any fruit, or vegetable, rich in vitamin C, appears to have a marked effect on cerebrovascular disease and hypertension, as a whole.

The reliance on the 'four basic foods' is an old fashioned, outdated and for many people, harmful hypothesis. We are all uniquely and biochemically different. For many, food from at least, two of the 'four' may cause a deterioration in health and loss of the ability to enjoy life — due to one, or more, of a wide range of chronic and debilitating symptoms. A final illustration comes in the form of a paragraph from Ross Horne's *New Health Revolution*:

In 1978 John Marino of Santa Monica, set a new USA cross country bicycle record of 13 days, 1 hour and 20 minutes. In 1979 on a diet high in rice and wheat, he tried to better that record, but could not complete the ride due to dizziness and fatigue and later found that he was allergic to these foods. In 1980 on a diet of fruit, vegetables, beans and fish, he knocked over 21 hours off his 1978 record to create a new one of 12 days, 3 hours and 41 minutes, and said he felt he could have continued riding, perhaps even back to Santa Monica.

Food additives

Amongst other things, food additives can cause skin allergies, according to an Atlanta dermatologist, Dr Richard Sturm. He has found that urticaria, a common symptom amongst food allergy sufferers, was caused by such additives as artificial colourings, tartrazine and sodium benzoate. Urticaria, incidentally, is the medical term for hives and produces swelling, puffiness, redness and itching. He found, also, that naturally occurring substances, such as yeast, benzoate and salicylate, were also implicated.

In Chapter 9, some mention was made of the great variety of chemicals used in our food today. There are now 5,000 different synthetic chemicals available in our daily diet and the average person consumes more than 3 kilos of these chemicals every year. It is no wonder that the body is becoming intolerant and rebelling. The human body simply cannot tolerate all these additional chemicals. It stops functioning properly, and becomes allergic and sick.

There is very strong evidence to support the fact that, damage is being done to people, by chemical additives that were previously thought to be safe. For example, saccharin is now banned in some countries, as it has been shown to cause bladder cancer, yet here in Australia it is still used freely in processed low calorie food and drinks. Other examples of harmful additives are monosodium glutemate (MSG) which can cause brain damage; brominated vegetable oil (BVO) which can lead to degeneration of the heart and testicles; ammoniated glycyrrhizin (licorice flavouring), a cause of high blood pressure. Some other common food additives considered to be dangerous are propylene glycol monostearate, butylated hydroxyanisole (BHA), butylated hydroxytoluene (BHT), carob bean gum, gum tragacanth, benzoic acid and sodium benzoate. If you don't believe these chemicals are in your food, start reading the extra fine print on labels. You might get a shock!

Choice magazine has advised parents against feeding their children with several well-known brands of breakfast cereal, as they contain the artificial colouring, tartrazine. Another source says that, in the United States alone, it is estimated that more than one million people are allergic to tartrazine, and it could be closer to ten million. Other dangerous additives mentioned were, sunset yellow, erythrocine and brilliant blue. These food colour chemicals are now known to cause allergies and hyperactivity. *Choice* also commented on the dangerous additives that are still to be found in Australian ice cream. These are:

Amaranth (red colouring), which was banned in the United States in 1976 when the Food and Drug Administration found it caused allergic reactions.

Carmosine, brilliant scarlet and chocolate brown colourings. These are banned in the Unites States, but still used in the United Kingdom and other EEC countries.

Brilliant blue is known to cause allergic responses, yet is still used in the United States and United Kingdom.

Chlorazol pink is banned in the United States, United Kingdom and EEC but still allowed in Australia.

Indigo carmine is currently under suspicion in the United States.

Sunset yellow and tartrazine, known to be widely allergenic, and, yet, still in use in the United States and Australia!

The odds are that, in time, most chemical additives will be proven harmful and banned. In the meantime, a lot of people are getting sick due to the massive toxic overload that these chemicals are causing in their bodies. If you want to get well, have healthy unclogged cells and be free from toxins and allergy illness, the message is clear — stay away from unnatural, potentially lethal, food additive chemicals.

Sugar

Sugar is the king of junk foods. It has absolutely no nutritional value, and today it is one of the most harmful substances known to man. It is particularly dangerous to people who are intolerant to refined grains and other carbohydrates. These people often suffer from hypoglycaemia, which is a distressing food allergy symptom. They are particularly affected by the fact that, when sugar is eaten, the result is a rapid rise, then a rapid fall, in blood sugar levels. Research has shown that this can cause extreme tiredness, marked irritability, aggressive behaviour, depression and a state of confusion.

It has also been indicated through research that sugar robs the body of zinc, thus affecting a variety of biochemical functions and particularly, the absorption of nutrients. This is because zinc is needed to activate some sixty enzyme systems in the body, and these are vital to proper digestion and absorption. In a recent study of 500 people in Perth, Western Australia, 70 per cent were found to be deficient in zinc!

The internationally renowned Canadian nutritionist, Dr Abraham Hoffer, points out that primitive tribes developed major health problems, within a mere twenty years of adopting a white man's diet. Along with other leading nutritionists, such as Nathan Pritikin and Drs Mackarness and Mindell, he cites sugar as being a major problem.

In 1300, when sugar was first introduced to Europe from India, a pound of sugar would have cost today's equivalent of $10,000. By 1850, sugar was cheap, and by 1975 it had become the most commonly used chemical in the processing of food. In the sixteenth century, people ate about 2 kilos of sugar per head, per year. Today, this has risen to a massive 60 kilos per year, in most Western countries.

Because of its extremely harmful effect on the pancreas, by stimulating overproduction of insulin, regular sugar intake causes allergic cravings for a variety of other, over-refined, junk foods. This, in turn, causes further deterioration in health and the development of further allergy addiction/illness. Combine this with its effect on the nutrient absorption process, and you have a permanent ticket to sickness and misery.

Avoid sugar — particularly in its most insidious form in processed foods. It has no nutritional content at all. It is totally unnecessary, extremely harmful and potentially lethal.

Dietary fibre

Much has been said about high fibre diets in the past few years, and there is no doubt that adequate fibre is necessary for good health. Unfortunately, the 'high fibre' approach is in danger of becoming a harmful fad as more and more people see it as the 'antidote' to their unhealthy eating habits. As with anything else, too much fibre can be harmful to health. Food needs a certain time to pass through the intestine so that vital nutrients can be absorbed by the body. If food is pushed through too fast, by unusually large intakes of fibre, the body does not get its full share of nutrients and can become undernourished. In other words, a form of malnutrition occurs. Zinc, in particular, has been found deficient in people on high fibre diets. This mineral is responsible for more functions than any other nutrient in the human body. Enzyme production, in particular, is affected by zinc deficiency. This is a very real problem and, as we have seen, lack of essential nutrients makes it impossible for the immune system to function properly.

A further trap for food allergy sufferers is that large intakes of unrefined cereal products are recommended in all high fibre diets. We now know that a very large number of people suffer, unknowingly, from intolerance and allergy to these foods. For these people, a deterioration in health will follow if excessive cereal/grain products are added to their diet.

The message is — be cautious of becoming too enthusiastically involved with the 'high fibre' philosophy. Occasional roughage, in the form of bran, wholemeal, etc., is fine if you are tolerant. Irrespective, it is more desirable to obtain sufficient fibre from other sources, such as peas, beans, nuts, dried fruit, desiccated coconut, lentils, apples, oranges and other fruits or vegetables.

Tea and coffee

Two words of warning on these appealing drinks. Drink sparingly!

Coffee, in particular, should not be drunk daily. It is just too harmful to the human system. However, like most things, there has to be a balance between doing harm to oneself and enjoying life. Although I am sensitive to coffee, I enjoy two or three cups per week. That way I don't feel too deprived, and the allergic effects are minimal. Coffee, on a regular basis, would poison me.

Earlier in this chapter, reference was made to research done at Sydney Hospital, indicating that a third of Australians are addicted to caffeine and only 3 per cent are strict abstainers, yet there is increasing evidence to show that caffeine causes disease! It is known that caffeine excites the nervous system, causes the kidneys to lose fluid and overworks the heart. It is also suspected of contributing to cancer, heart attack and stroke. It is basically a poison and, taken regularly, can lead to allergy addiction and toxic overload.

Decaffeinated coffee, unfortunately, is not any safer. *Choice* magazine recently referred to the chemical trichloroethylene, a toxic substance similar to drycleaning fluid, which was previously used in the decaffeination process. Evidently, because of its toxicity, it has been superseded by another chemical, methylene chloride. However, tests at the United States Community Nutrition Institute, show that this chemical causes cancer, so it's a case of the caffeine being replaced by another harmful substance. It would seem sensible to view decaffeinated coffee with extreme caution.

According to nutrition author, Dr Earl Mindell, while the average cup of instant coffee has 66 mg of caffeine, percolated and drip-method coffees have a massive 146 mg per cup. Evidently, the longer the coffee is in contact with the water, the greater the caffeine content. It is interesting to note that cola has 64.7 mg, per 340 ml can, which is only slightly less than a cup of instant coffee.

So much for coffee. What about tea? The only difference between tea and coffee is caffeine content. Whilst the average cup of instant coffee has 66 mg, a cup of tea has about 46 mg. Therefore, it will take an equivalent quantity of tea about 50 per cent longer, to do the same toxic job on you than coffee. If you brew your own coffee and drink an equivalent number of cups, per day, you will get sick three times faster than a tea drinker.

If you are in good health, and free from toxic overload, two or three cups of tea, per day, should not be a problem, as the body's normal detoxification processes can handle it. However, if you are on an average Australian diet, beware! The odds are your detoxification processes are already working overtime.

Alcohol

Alcohol should be avoided whenever possible. All alcohol contains yeast and other allergens from the base ingredients, such as grains and malt. If you do drink alcohol regularly, remember it should be treated in the same manner as other food substances. Firstly, it should be taken in moderation and not more than once every four days, (Four-day-rotation diet). Secondly, if you do drink it more than once in a four-day period, switch to a different form, to avoid over-exposure to the same allergen. For example, alternate between beer and wine. Avoid red wines because of their high histamine content. Dry white wine and well watered white spirits are the least harmful if drunk in moderation.

Eating habits to promote good health

Eat only when hungry This is difficult for people with addictive food allergies, because of the artificial hunger pangs caused by this problem. Hunger should be a comfortable feeling, resulting from the body needing food for energy, rather than from the ravenous cravings, caused by food allergy.

Eat slowly and relax Remember, saliva contains digestive enzymes. Thorough chewing considerably aids digestion and assimilation of food. Food broken down into fine particles by plenty of chewing, places much less strain on the digestive system.

Eat small meals It is better to eat five, or six, small meals per day, than three larger ones. The 'three meals per day' habit is like the 'four basic foods' idea — a fallacy! If you eat smaller meals, your digestive system is not overloaded and, thus, operates more efficiently, nutrient absorption is much better and fat assimilation is less.

Do not eat too many foods at once The fewer foods you eat at one meal, the better. Digestion and nutrient absorption is far more efficient. This is one reason why primitive races do not suffer from indigestion and flatulence. They extract maximum nutrients from very simple diets.

Do not mix raw fruits and vegetables Both raw fruits and raw vegetables should be eaten separately. The same applies to juices. The reason is that totally different enzymes are needed to digest each one. Thus, if you mix them up, poor digestion and flatulence will follow. Remember, poor digestion and assimilation stimulates allergy problems and is the root cause of many illnesses.

Always eat protein foods last Proteins require a generous amount of hydrochloric acid, in the stomach, to enable the enzymes to break them down effectively. This process takes about twice as long as that of carbohydrates. When these are eaten, little hydrochloric acid is secreted, as carbohydrates do not need much for digestion. Accordingly, they tend to pass much quicker into the duodenum. However, if carbohydrates are eaten after protein, they are held back in the stomach, by the protein, and fermentation commences.

This affects the digestion of carbohydrates and the assimilation of nutrients. It slows the passage of carbohydrates through the system, increases the absorption of toxins and creates elimination problems for the colon.

Undereat whenever possible A major study of centenarians, of greatly diverse backgrounds, produced one common denominator. They all ate sparingly, throughout their lives! Systematic undereating is the greatest single aid to good health. Even the best possible diet, eaten to excess, will lead to food intolerances and degenerative disease. Over indulgence in high protein foods is especially harmful. Light meals lead to better digestion, greater utilisation of nutrients and, believe it or not, fewer hunger pangs.

Do not drink with meals Although a glass of wine occasionally is harmless, generally, drinking with meals, or immediately before or after meals, should be avoided. The dilution of essential hydrochloric acid in the stomach, can have a detrimental effect on efficient digestion and absorption.

This chapter is best summed up by comments from two leading American nutrition experts. Dr John Douglas, of the Kaiser Medical Centre, in Los Angeles, says:

1 Eat foods as close to their natural state as possible
2 Eat a lot of your foods uncooked
3 Eat foods you control, not foods that control you. If you love it — or hate it, avoid it.

Furthermore, according to Dr Frederick Trowbridge, of the Centre for Disease Control, Atlanta, malnutrition is rife amongst overfed Western civilisation. He says, overeating of too much over-refined processed junk, is causing grave nutrient deficiencies, leading to ecological illness and disease in people of all ages.

Food sources of nutrients

Vitamin A

Beef liver	Swordfish	Carrots
Halibut	Spinach	Tomato
Salmon	Beet greens	Kale
Cream cheese	Mustard greens	Sweet potato
Mackerel	Squash	Melons
Crab	Grapefruit	Papaya
Oysters		

Vitamin C

Beef liver	Tomato	Avocado
Oysters	Broccoli	Blackberries
Brazil nuts	Cabbage	Cherries
Potato	Spinach	Raspberries
Squash	Collard	Blueberries
Sweet potato	Citrus fruit	Banana
Alfalfa sprouts	Cantaloupe	Pineapple
Mustard greens	Rosehips	Gooseberries
Green pepper	Strawberries	

Vitamin D

Beef liver	Tuna	Chicken liver
Sardines	Milk	Herring
Salmon	Egg Yolk	

Vitamin E

Cold-pressed oils	Parsley	Wheat germ
Eggs	Sweet potato	

Vitamin F

Vegetable oils	Butter	Sunflower seeds

Vitamin K

Liver	Soy	Cauliflower
Egg yolk	Broccoli	Green leafy vegetables

Thiamine B-1

Beef heart	Mackerel	Pumpkin
Beef liver	Perch	Soy
Beef kidney	Red Snapper	Pork liver
Milk	Wheat	Brazil nuts

Crab
Oysters
Cod
Trout
Flounder

Rice
Barley
Pineapple
Peanuts
Pumpkin

Cashews
Pecans
Sesame seeds
Sunflower seeds

Riboflavin B-2

Beef
Beef kidney
Beef heart
Beef liver
Chicken liver
Trout

Cod
Mackerel
Perch
Clams
Oysters

Salmon
Collard
Mushrooms
Brazil nuts
Almonds

Pyridoxine B-6

Beef
Beef liver
Beef heart
Chicken
Milk
Halibut
Mackerel
Salmon

Sardines
Tuna
Crab
Pork liver
Pork heart
Barley
Wheat
Rice

Prunes
Avocado
Brazil nuts
Peanuts
Peas
Soy
Lentils
Lima beans

B-12

Beef
Beef liver
Pork liver
Milk

Cheddar cheese
Cream cheese
Yoghurt
Sardines

Tuna
Egg
Prunes

B-15

Apricot kernels
Rice bran

Rice shoots
Brewer's yeast

Liver

Niacin

Beef
Beef liver
Beef kidney
Chicken
Turkey
Pork
Clams
Oysters

Halibut
Haddock
Strawberries
Raspberries
Squash
Tomato
Potato
Broccoli

Avocado
Papaya
Watermelon
Soy
Wheat
Barley
Rice
Corn

Crab
Shrimp
Cod
Perch
Trout
Salmon
Mackerel
Sardines

Collard
Mushrooms
Green beans
Lima beans
Garbanzo beans
Peas
Dried apricots
Peaches

Peanuts
Almonds
Pumpkin seeds
Sunflower seeds
Pecans
Cashews
Brazil nuts
Boysenberries

Folic Acid

Beef liver
Beef heart
Turkey
Cottage cheese
Mackerel
Tuna

Barley
Rice
Peanuts
Lima beans
Blackberries
Avocado

Plums
Raisins
Almonds
Pecans
Walnuts
Dates

Pantothenic Acid

Beef
Beef liver
Pork liver
Chicken
Salmon
Mackerel

Sardines
Lobster
Clams
Crab
Mushrooms
Avocado

Watermelon
Pineapple
Soy
Lentils
Bean sprouts
Peanuts

Inositol

Beef
Beef liver
Pork
Chicken

Rice
Peanuts
Apple
Grapefruit

Orange
Raisins
Strawberries
Salmon

Choline

Beef
Beef liver
Pork liver
Milk

Egg
Split peas
Peanuts
Soy

Green beans
Bean sprouts
Garbanzo beans
Lentils

Biotin

Beef
Beef liver
Pork liver
Chicken
Eggs

Salmon
Lima beans
Split peas
Turnip greens
Cauliflower

Peanuts
Soy
Avocado
Grapefruit
Watermelon

Sardines	Mushrooms	Almonds
Mackerel	Garbanzo beans	Pecans
Tuna	Lentils	

Rutin

Buckwheat	Liver	Eggs

Para-aminobenzoic Acid (PABA)

Beef liver	Beef kidney	Wheatgerm
Beef heart	Yoghurt	Green leafy vegetables

Bio-flavinoids

Lemon	Grapefruit	Red pepper
Lime	Orange	

Zinc

Oysters	Grains	Pork
Pumpkin seeds	Sunflower seeds	Beef liver

Manganese

Egg yolk	Nuts	Sunflower seeds
Grain	Pineapple	

Magnesium

Beef	Crab	Avocado
Milk	Shrimp	Dates
Pork	Barley	Pecans
Chicken	Rice	Almonds
Salmon	Peanuts	Cashews
Flounder	Sesame	Brazil nuts
Tuna	Dried apricots	

Potassium

Beef	Perch	Dates
Beef liver	Clams	Papaya
Milk	Tomato	Avocado
Turkey	Collard	Apricots
Pork	Lima beans	Bananas
Sardines	Split peas	Brazil nuts
Cod	Peanuts	Pecans
Flounder	Soy	Almonds

Haddock	Sunflower seeds	Orange
Salmon		

Calcium

Beef liver	Crab	Turnip greens
Chicken liver	Oysters	Collard
Milk	Shrimp	Mustard greens
Yoghurt	Mackerel	Sesame seeds
Cheese	Sardines	Brazil nuts
Clams	Salmon	Almonds

Phosphorus

Beef	Mackerel	Rice
Beef liver	Sardines	Peanuts
Pork liver	Clams	Barley
Chicken	Cod	Sunflower seeds
Turkey	Haddock	Sesame seeds
Eggs	Perch	Pecans
Oysters	Tuna	Walnuts
Milk	Shrimp	Cashews
Yoghurt	Lobster	Almonds
Cheese	Crab	Brazil nuts
Salmon	Flounder	Soy

Iron

Beef	Flounder	Garbanzo beans
Beef liver	Haddock	Lima beans
Beef kidney	Mackerel	Soy
Pork	Perch	Raisins
Pork liver	Tuna	Prunes
Chicken	Salmon	Brazil nuts
Clams	Wheat	Sunflower seeds
Oysters	Dried apricots	Walnuts
Shrimp	Eggplant	Sesame seeds
Sardines	Tomato	Almonds
Cod	Pumpkin seeds	Peanuts

Iodine

Salmon	All oils	Butter
Turkey	Shredded wheat	Lard
Rabbit		

Copper

Calf liver	Mushrooms	Pork liver
Lamb liver	Sunflower seeds	Brazil nuts
Oysters	Yeast	Filberts
Wheatgerm	Tea	Walnuts

Molybdenum

Buckwheat	Wheatgerm	Lentils
Eggs	Lima beans	Sunflower seeds
Oats	Barley	Liver
Soybean		

Selenium

| Garlic | Brown rice | Eggs |
| Brewer's yeast | Liver | |

Chromium

Eggs	Brewer's yeast	Mushrooms
Beets	Whole wheat bread	Liver
Molasses	Black pepper	Beef

NUTRIENT THERAPY

A key to good health

What is a nutrient? The *World Book Dictionary* defines a nutrient as 'a nourishing substance, especially as an element or ingredient of a foodstuff'. It is derived from the Latin word, nutriens, as is nutrition — which means 'the process, by which living things take in food and use it'. In the normal scheme of things, we eat a balanced diet, and from the diet come all the various chemical components that the body needs for efficient functioning. This is assuming that the body's own chemical machinery is intact and in perfect working order.

What happens when the body is not in perfect working order? When, in fact, the chemical mechanisms, that are supposed to keep the body in this state, are defective and have always been so? This condition is not evident and the individual looks normal. Physical defects are patently obvious, but it is not possible to know, just by looking at a person, whether or not his cell structure is defective.

In reality, medical practice is still at a fairly basic stage. It concentrates its approach on the obvious and, doggedly, persists in treating symptoms with drugs, without searching for the underlying cause. Drugs, being alien chemicals, are not, normally, present in the human body cells. They interfere dramatically with man's biochemistry and do not prevent the disease process. At best, they offer symptomatic relief, whilst the causal process continues, uninterrupted. This approach is totally wrong. Apart from surgical

173

procedures, such as those to repair deformities and injuries, modern medical practice is often inefficient and harmful. The compulsive prescription of drugs is doing constant harm to the very people they are supposed to be helping. The result is further damage to body chemistry which is already malfunctioning.

A newspaper article on Lady Phyllis Cilento, quoted her as saying:

The whole of the medical profession is being run by the drug companies. The drug companies dare not acknowledge vitamins—they are too cheap. Their patent, expensive drugs would become redundant. Vitamin C is the only effective antibiotic against virus, the only one that can detoxify and stimulate the immune system.

The article explained that she was on a strong daily programme of vitamin C, vitamin E and multiple vitamins and minerals. She has almost finished her fifteenth book and is halfway through her autobiography. Although Lady Cilento is ninety-one years of age, she still sees patients in her downstairs surgery. If her example is not a testimony to the merits of daily nutrient supplements, I don't know what else could be.

It should be understood that the body is nothing more, or less, than a chemical factory, although its chemical complexity is still largely beyond human comprehension. Our movements, our senses, and, to some extent, our thoughts, are generated by myriad flash-like chemical reactions, which send impulses at lightning speed throughout the body. These reactions originate in the body's cells, each an individual mechanism in its own right, a billion times more complex than the most complex computer ever devised.

A person born without an arm, or a leg, is unlucky, but, nevertheless is aware of the defect because it is obvious. That person can still go on to lead a vigorous life, within certain limitations. But what about a person born with a defective cell structure? In other words, something is missing, just as a limb may be missing. He cannot see himself as restricted because, as far as he is aware, he is not. Why? Because it is not possible to look at a cell, except through a microscope, and even then, what can be seen is extremely limited. Modern medical science cannot, yet, look at a cell, (of which there are ten million, million, in the human body), and ascertain whether all of its myriad functions are operating properly. This relates particularly to the ability of each cell to successfully process and/ or manufacture, the forty or so nutrients vital for optimum health. In this respect detailed scientific knowledge of the working of the human cell, has barely scratched the surface.

However, some extremely good guesswork, initially, followed by practical trials in thousands of clinical cases, has shown that genetic defects do exist in many individuals. These defects can affect cell activity to a point where the individual never knows what it is like to experience a normal health state. The results of such defects are, in fact, catastrophic—certainly far more devastating than the absence of an arm or leg. Often the individual endures a lifetime of pain, suffering and mental illness, the cause of which remains undetected and generally unsuspected by the conventional medical practitioner.

You may well ask why this is so when a number of books, based on a great many case histories, have been published in America over the past ten years. Such eminent people as Professor Linas Pauling (twice Nobel Prize winner), Dr William Philpott, Dr Theron Randolph, Dr Roger Williams, Dr H. J. Rinkel, Dr W. C. Alverez and many, many others, have published excellent detailed and authoritative works on their successes in the use of the orthomolecular approach. These eminent doctors can refer to many thousands of cases where mental illness, autism, and multiple allergy conditions, have been rectified by the use of selective food avoidance and nutrient therapy. Unfortunately, many medical practitioners are stereotyped in their thinking and remain conservative people who tend to reject change. The suffering caused in our society, by this narrow-minded approach, is tragic. Time and time again, people affected by food and chemical allergies have been classified by the doctors as 'neurotic' or 'phsychologically unsound'. Such a gross display of ignorance by a, supposedly, compassionate body of people is inexcusable. The medical profession, in general, has shown an inability to cope with the unknown. Many doctors find it impossible to accept that they should have to look beyond their individual fund of knowledge to find the cause of a patient's distress. As a result, they have never heard of the doctors previously mentioned, nor read any of their works. This is a tragic situation which must not be allowed to continue.

One such book that all doctors should read is *Brain Allergies the Psychonutrient Connection*, written by Drs William Philpott and Dwight Kalita. They make the fundamental point that orthomolecular (nutrient) therapy is far superior to toximolecular (drug) therapy, because it recognises that a healthy body must have healthy cells. The aim of the orthomolecular physician is, therefore, to ensure that all cells have the correct proportions of the very things on which their existence depends. These are vitamins, minerals, amino acids, etc. and are referred to collectively as nutrients.

Doctors who are interested in curing and preventing the causes of disease, rather than merely relieving symptoms, must make use of the orthomolecular approach. There is no other way to stem the ever-increasing tide of chronic illness and degenerative disease. Otherwise, the Western world in particular, is just going to get sicker. According to Drs Philpott and Kalita, statistical analysis in America indicates that unless doctors change their ways, the medical field will grow from being the third largest industry, to the largest industry in the country. Furthermore, by the year 2000, it would require the entire gross national product to support it.

Orthomolecular medicine

This term was first used by Professor Linus Pauling in 1968. It means, literally, 'pertaining to the right molecule'. Orthomolecular physicians believe that by increasing or varying the concentration of 'right molecules' in the body, infections and degenerative diseases can be successfully treated. The 'right molecules' are the vitamins, minerals, trace elements, amino acids, enzymes and hormones which are normally present in the human body. The concept of orthomolecular medicine begins with the cell itself. The belief is, that if the nutritional balance of each body cell is correct, then optimum health is maintained. On the other hand, nutritional deficiencies in the cells constitute the major cause of disease. The orthomolecular approach aims at providing each and every cell of our bodies with optimum nutrients, so that proper and healthy functioning is ensured. The individual's internal environment then remains in biochemical harmony and chronic and degenerative disease cannot take hold.

The list of necessary nutrients is the same for every human being, but the relative amounts needed by each individual are different. This is because the kind of food you eat, the physical, mental and emotional stress you experience, the environment you live and work in, the exercise you do and so on, even down to the type of water you drink, all add up to a picture of the individual. Combine these factors with your inherited biochemical make-up, and you become a 'one off' with unique biochemical needs. Many illnesses occur because the body cells are ailing, as they are not being adequately provided with the optimum nutrients that are needed to sustain, and propagate, healthy tissues and organs.

Often, this can happen on the best of healthy diets. Why? Because many individuals, due to genetic biochemical defects, are not able to absorb, or metabolise, the necessary nutrients from food which their body needs to sustain health. Allergy sufferers, inevitably, fit into this group. The most chronic sufferers of multiple allergy illness will receive great benefit from a carefully contrived regimen of nutrients, taken daily. Through testing and retesting, orthomolecular physicians are able to arrive, eventually, at the appropriate nutrients and dosages required for each person. It is not uncommon to find that an individual needs massive doses of some nutrients to balance his chemical structure—perhaps up to one hundred times the average daily amount. In reality 'average' intake is a fallacy. Because each person is biochemically unique, daily requirements can vary enormously from person to person, particularly when someone is born with biochemically defective cells. About the average person, Dr Vayda says:

The concept of the average person is a laboratory inspired one, and very useful to scientists because they need to have nice neat statistics so that they can do proper research. But can their statistics help you? In the field of nutrition they're some use, but often they make as much sense as trying to fit all women into an average size bra . . . they can be misleading when applied to individuals as the statistician found out when he tried to cross a river with an average depth of three feet and drowned in the section where it was twenty-five feet deep.

In other words, Dr Vayda is saying what Dr Philpott and others are

177

saying: vitamin, mineral, amino acid etc, requirements can vary enormously from person to person. Remember, you may not be an average person. If your cells require an unusually large amount of a particular nutrient to stay healthy, and you are not getting it, you are in trouble. In fact, you are sitting in a chemical powder keg. It is only a matter of time before the body cells begin to deteriorate, resulting in chemical intolerance to a range of foods and other substances.

Orthomolecular physicians have had spectacular success, in the past few years, in rectifying allergy illness by the use of nutrient supplements, together with dietary control; that is, identification and avoidance of major allergens. It has been found that the use of nutrient supplements will provide resistance to allergenic food, so that some tolerance may be acquired. This is certainly a great 'plus' for the sufferer, if it means he can sometimes eat his favourite foods without getting sick. Believe me, it is marvellous!

Toximolecular medicine

This is a common type of therapy, involving the use of drugs at sub-lethal levels. It has been used by physicians for only about forty years. Drugs, being alien chemicals, radically alter the biochemical environment inside the human body, and often cause very serious and dangerous side effects. Often, with drug therapy, it is a matter of using a 'sledgehammer to crack a walnut'. Writing about this, Dr Philpott explains 'drugs do not halt or prevent the disease process, especially degenerative disease; at best they offer symptomatic relief, while the fundamental underlying disease process continues uninterrupted'.

Dr Roger J. Williams writes on drugs, in his book, *Nutrition against Disease*:

> They have no connection with the disease process itself . . . they tend to mask the difficulty, not eliminate it. They contaminate the internal environment (with side effects) create dependence on the part of the patient and often complicate the physician's job by erasing valuable clues as to the real source of trouble.

It is obvious what these physicians think of drug therapy. Yet, this is the most common form of medicine practised in the world today.

The allergy sufferer gains absolutely nothing from a constant stream of drugs, supplied by doctors to fix his symptoms. Drugs do not fix symptoms, they *mask* symptoms and further weaken the immune system. On the other hand, orthomolecular medicine seeks to boost the immune system, by giving it the essential nutrients to help it do its job—that of overcoming disease and restoring chemical balance to the body. There is only one healer and that is the body itself. Natural substances, such as vitamins, minerals, amino acids, enzymes, etc., introduced to the body in proper doses, help the body heal itself, because they are what the body lives on. Drugs, on the other hand, are completely foreign substances and invariably result in further damage to the immune system, due to side effects and toxic overload.

Figures produced in America, a few years ago, showed that, in one year, the population swallowed 700,909 kilos of tranquillizers, 380,000 kilos of barbiturates and 1,835,000 kilos of penicillin; yet 93 million of 213 million people, almost half the population, suffered from some form of degenerative disease. These statistics have since become worse. Obviously, symptomatic drug therapy is a dismal failure.

Although some of the resource material contained in this book comes from non-medical people, most of the researchers and authors quoted are qualified medical practitioners, who have realized that the drug approach is simply not the answer. They know all about drug therapy because they were taught it at University, during their medical course. However, realizing how futile and harmful drug therapy has become, they have virtually started again and evolved treatment processes that are, not only safe for the body, but also effective. They have not gone to all this extra trouble for nothing. It would have been easy for them to have sat in their offices, like their average counterpart, and dispensed prescriptions. But too many people were suffering as a result of that dubious approach, and, fortunately, a few doctors cared enough to look for better methods. This resulted in the birth, in recent years, of alternative forms of medicine, which have proven to be highly successful. Orthomolecular medicine has only been followed in Australia in the past two or three years. The successes enjoyed by the doctors who are practising this form of medicine will force the traditional, drug-oriented doctor to change his thinking as more time goes by. The real change will take place when the nation's medical schools change their philosophy.

The plain truth is that the orthomolecular approach can greatly assist allergy sufferers to regain good health, whereas the toximolecular approach is virtually useless. It has been estimated that 20 per cent of the population suffers from masked or multiple allergy illness, to some degree, so there is an enormous number of people who are not being helped at all by the current medical approach. As Dr Philpott says:

> The field of allergies is much larger than traditional immunologists have claimed. There are many maladaptive, allergic-like reactions, including central nervous system reactions, that do not manifest antibody formation and therefore, do not fit the immunologists narrow definition of allergy.

Supernutrition — The orthomolecular approach

Supernutrition is based on the fact that, apart from an ample supply of water and oxygen, a team of about forty nutrients, combined in just the right proportions, is essential for the maintenance of optimum health in each cell of the body. Unless the diet contains adequate amounts of these nutrients, and the body is able to absorb them in sufficient quantities, it is impossible to maintain good health.

For the many reasons, referred to in early chapters, our body cells often have to put up with environments that fall far short of the ideal. They become clogged with chemicals and miscellaneous rubbish that impairs their ability to function properly. This, in turn, leads to a wide range of health problems and an inability to process nutrients effectively. The situation is often further aggravated by damage to the system, such as intestinal damage, which make the digestion, absorption and transportation of nutrients inefficient. Thus, the cells do not receive all of their essential requirements. If the cell itself is genetically defective, resulting in an impaired ability to metabolise a certain vitamin, or produce a particular enzyme, then you have a further cause of nutrient deficiency.

Thus, for a variety of reasons, your body may need more of a particular nutrient, or even more of most nutrients, than a person without these problems; and if you don't get them, you become ill and stay ill. Some people are never well, right from infancy. Others, due to environmental factors, develop nutrient deficiencies during adulthood, which cause a progressive decline in their health because the body ceases to function properly. It develops allergies and intolerances, accumulates toxic waste matter and vital functions being to deteriorate. A wide range of chronic and debilitating symptoms develop which make life a continual misery. Finally, the toxic overload becomes concentrated in a vital organ, or other bodily system, and your doctor diagnoses a diseased kidney, multiple sclerosis or whatever, and sets about treating what is really only a symptom of nutritional deficiency. Surgery, or toximolecular therapy, may actually arrest the manifestation of your illness, in that particular direction. But what about the cause (nutritional deficiency) associated with toxic overload from food and chemical sensitivities? The cause is usually overlooked. Although some attention may be paid to diet, this is rarely enough. Inevitably, the person concerned will develop another disease and, finally the body will give up the struggle. Either that, or they will linger on, year after year, too drugged, sick and tired to enjoy full potential of life.

In the case of chronic illness, such as suffered by those allergic to foods and chemicals, nutrient therapy can be extremely helpful. My own experiences have confirmed the validity of the orthomolecular approach. I take a range of nutrients daily. This coupled with sensible avoidance of personal allergens, has resulted in the space of a few months, in a change from chronic ill heath to an excellent level of good health and energy. For me, nutrient therapy has played a major role in my recovery from a wide range of symptoms, both physical and mental, that had baffled the medical profession since I was an infant.

Studies undertaken at the University of California, Los Angeles School of Medicine, have found that the average daily diet is particularly lacking in zinc, vitamin E, copper, magnesium, iron, niacin, vitamin B-12, pantothenic acid, calcium, riboflavin, folate, vitamins A, B-6, B-1 and vitamin C. Although this information is not necessarily relevant to everyone, (considering Dr Vayda's comments on the term 'average'), it does serve to illustrate that nutrient deficiency is a fact of life, and each of us should be aware of the varying effects it can have on our individual health.

Nutrient therapy

Dr R. J. Williams, in *Nutrition Against Disease*, has formulated a basic nutrient programme for people who do not suffer from allergic, or addictive, responses to food and chemicals. He suggests the following doses:

Vitamin A	7500 IU	Para-aminobenzoic Acid (PABA)	30 mg
D	400 IU	Rutin	200 mg
E	40 IU	Calcium	750 mg
K	2 mg	Phosphate	750 mg
C	250 mg	Magnesium	200 mg
B-1	2 mg	Iron	15 mg
B-2	2 mg	Zinc	15 mg
B-6	3 mg	Copper	2 mg
B-12	9 mcg	Iodine	0.15 mg
Niacinamide	20 mg	Manganese	5 mg
Biotin	0.3 mg	Molybdenum	0.1 mg
Folic Acid	0.4 mg	Chromium	1.0 mg
Choline	250 mg	Selenium	0.02 mg
Inositol	250 mg	Cobalt	0.1 mg
Pantothenic Acid	15 mg		

According to Dr Williams, the daily intake of these nutrients should give a considerable degree of protection against the development of food and chemical allergy illness. Although the list looks formidable, most of these nutrients can be taken in the form of a few multi-vitamin and multi-mineral pills each day. He suggests a rotational approach to foods which means not eating the same foods every day but rather every few days.

According to Dr Lendon Smith in his book *Feed Yourself Right*, poor nutrition is one of the major causes of health problems. He offers a daily basic nutrient programme as follows:

Vitamin A	10,000 to 20,000 IU
B complex	50 mg of each B Vitamin
B-12	100 mcg
Choline	1000 mg
Inositol	1000 mg
Pantothenic acid	50 to 100 mg
Folic acid	0.4 mg
C	1000 to 5000 mg or more
D	500 to 1000 IU — depending on sun exposure
E	400 IU
Calcium	500 to 1000 mg
Magnesium	300 to 500 mg

Trace elements — especially chromium, selenium and zinc.

Dr Smith makes mention of the need to make adjustments for your age, he says that vitamin C, and B-complex, are particularly important for those over forty. Those over fifty need more B6, while those over seventy require more vitamin A. However, when chronic physical problems are present, indicating allergy illness, much larger doses of nutrients are required. These should always be tailored, where possible, by an orthomolecular practitioner, to suit the needs of the individual. Dr Philpott suggests daily dosages, within the following ranges, depending on severity of illness:

Vitamin A	10,000 to 50,000 IU
B-1	100 to 1,500 mg
B-2	100 to 1,500 mg
B-12	500 to 3,000 mcg
Niacin	200 to 1,500 mg
Biotin	0.3 to 0.6 mg
Choline	250 to 1,000 mg
Folic Acid	1 to 5 mg
Inositol	500 to 1000 mg

Para-Aminobenzoic Acid (PABA)	300 to 1,500 mg
Pantothenic Acid	100 to 1,500 mg
Vitamin C	1,000 to 10,000 mg or higher
D	400 to 1,200 IU
E	400 to 2,400 IU
Calcium	500 to 1,000 mg
Magnesium	100 to 300 mg
Iodine	150 to 300 mcg
Copper	5 to 15 mg
Zinc	15 to 30 mg
Chromium	1 to 3 mg
Manganese	5 to 15 mg
Selenium	200 mcg

At these levels it is best to consult a physician who specialises in the use of mega-vitamin therapy.

In recent years, researchers have found that the immune system needs a full supply of all nutrients to function efficiently. When it is under siege, from excessive body toxins, it is essential that supplements be added to the diet. Some examples are:

Vitamin A
According to New York State University, people taking a supplement of 5000 IU of vitamin A, per day, had half the developing cancer, compared with people taking 1700 IU per day. This was because vitamin A greatly improves the performance of the immune system and enables the body to deal more effectively with toxic overload.

Vitamin C
There is such a massive body of evidence to support the need for vitamin C supplement these days, that those who do not take it daily are throwing away the best opportunity ever, to improve their health. According to Dr Ringsdorf, of Sydney University, vitamin C greatly strengthens the immune system. A strong immune system will protect you from all manner of chronic allergy symptoms, of which the common cold is one of the most tedious. Dr Ringsdorf found that, in ninety-five pairs of identical twins, the twin given

1000 Mg of vitamin C, over a 100-day period, experienced fewer colds and they were less severe, than the other twin who was given a placebo.

Vitamin D

The International Journal for Vitamin and Nutrition Research has reported on research carried out on sixty-three elderly people in Sweden. It found that 30 per cent of these people had weak immune systems. Blood tests showed that most were deficient in vitamin D. After three months of vitamin D, and other supplements, their immune systems returned to normal.

Zinc

Research carried out at the University of Florida, by Dr Patricia Wagner, showed that 22 per cent of men and women, aged between sixty and ninety, had such low zinc levels that their immune systems were rendered ineffective. Zinc supplements, over a four-week period, raised immune resistance back to normal levels. According to *Prevention* magazine, zinc levels, in Western societies, can be so low that deficiency occurs within twenty-four hours of commencing a fast. Low zinc levels go with low iron and folic acid levels and, often, the most vulnerable person is the pregnant teenager. In these cases a deprived immune system can result in allergy responses developing in both mother and child.

Copper

According to Dr Leslie Klevay, of the Human Nutrition Research Centre in North Dakota, only about one quarter of human diets provide the minimum daily requirement of copper. He says that even a relatively mild copper deficiency leads to impaired sugar metabolism and high blood cholesterol. As we have previously seen, impaired ability to metabolise sugar, causes fermentation in the small intestine, which seriously affects digestion and absorption. Food intolerance and allergy reactions follow.

Selenium

Dr Stephen Levine of the Allergy Research Group, has found that selenium supplementation has totally reversed his own severe chemical hypersensitivities. He says that selenium supplements will improve chemical tolerance to phenols, formaldehyde, hydrocarbons and chlorine for many chemically allergic people. Evidently, selenium, like vitamin C, is a very effective anti-oxidant and anti-inflammatory agent.

Amino acids

In addition to vitamins, minerals and trace elements, equally important are amino acids and enzymes. As Dr Williams says:

> It must be emphasised that adequate nutrition must involve the complete chain of nutrients. If a diet is missing one link in the nutritional chain, it may be as worthless for supporting life as if it were missing ten links. One nutrient, i.e. mineral, amino acid or vitamin, added as a supplement to a food can bring no favourable effect unless the food contains all the other nutrients.

With respect to enzymes, reference should be made to Chapter 16 as this subject is important enough to merit being dealt with separately.

Amino acids should also be taken under the guidance of an orthomolecular physician, whenever possible, as this area of nutrient therapy requires a more specific approach. However, in general terms, great benefit can be gained by daily dosages of the following essential amino acids.

L–Arginine	L–Leucine
L–Histidine	L–Lysine
L–Isoleucine	L–Tyrosine
L–Methionine	L–Threonine
L–Phenylalanine	L–Valine
L–Tryptophan	

The essential amino acids are those which the body cannot itself produce and, under normal circumstances, are extracted from our diet. The 'non-essential amino acids', which under normal circumstances are produced by the body, may be just as important, however, because the body may not be functioning well enough to produce them in sufficient quantities. These are:

L–Alanine	L–Glycine
L–Aspartic Acid	L–Hydroxyproline
L–Cystine	L–Proline
L–Glutamic Acid	L–Serine

Here again, these lists appear to be formidable but, in reality, amino acid supplements are surprisingly easy to take. Bioglan Laboratories, an Australian company, has a superb range of all nutrients, including an amino acid complex capsule, which contains all of the essential, and most of the non-essential, amino acids.

According to Dr Stephen Levine, Director of the Allergy Research Group in California, amino acids in sufficient quantities cannot always be absorbed from a normal diet—even one high in protein. He says that it is quite clear that many of us suffer from amino acid deficiencies, particularly people with food and other addictions. In *Nutrition Against Disease,* Dr Roger Williams says:

> It should not be taken for granted, for example, that an individual getting plenty of good quality protein food is, *ipso facto,* well supplied with all the needed amino acids: but as we have seen, problems involving biochemical individuality in digestive (or absorptive) enzymes may intervene. Amino acids as such are available and can be supplied directly.

Amino acid deficiency is directly linked with pancreatic enzyme deficiency, brought about by food/chemical allergy addiction, according to Drs Philpott and Kalita. The resultant hypopancreatic function causes reduced production of protease enzymes, which are needed in the manufacture of amino acids. A further consequence of hypopancreatic function is a reduction in bicarbonate, which leads to destruction of proteolytic enzymes in the small intestine and, thus, further amino acid deficiencies.

Elderly people are particularly susceptible to amino acid deficiencies. Studies, in the *American Journal of Clinical Nutrition,* indicated that more than one third of men and women, over the age of sixty, had amino acid levels that were either deficient or low.

Dr Levine is adamant that amino acid supplementation will 'dramatically increase tolerance to previously hypersensitising foods and chemicals'. He reminds us that the forty or so, neurotransmitters are, themselves, mainly amino acids, or derived from amino acids. He further suggests that 'amino acid support for allergic individuals is critical and more effective than digestive enzyme therapy'.

According to the *Journal of Pharmaceutical Science*, when rats were given supplements of the amino acids tryptophan and lysine, they were protected from the intoxicating effects of both alcohol and barbiturates. Furthermore, sleeplessness, a common symptom amongst allergy sufferers, can be helped considerably, by taking 1500 Mg of L–Tryptophan at bedtime. This can be repeated after one hour, if necessary.

Hormones

According to Dr Philpott, the pancreas is not the only endocrine gland significantly involved in the degenerative disease process. He says, that allergy reactions to foods and chemicals, produce a situation in the body whereby the normal processes of all the glands are altered. As a result, either overproduction or underproduction of hormones occurs.

The endocrine glands are ductless glands which secrete hormones to influence other organs in the body. They are particularly concerned with the way the body uses food, so their stability and efficiency is vital to the allergy sufferer. They consist of the pineal, pituitary thyroid, thymus, pancreas, adrenals, ovaries and testes.

In severe cases, involving continuing underproduction of hormones, supplementary treatment may be required. This can only be prescribed by a medical doctor. Usually, avoidance of allergenic substances, plus nutrient supplements, will allow the endocrine glands, the pancreas, in particular, to regain proper function eventually. Attention should be paid, not only to supplements, but also to eating the right foods, in order to give the body maximum access to nutrients in their natural form. For this reason, careful note should be taken of the lists in Chapter 14, showing natural food sources of vitamins, minerals and trace elements. In the case of allergy illness, the body may be allergic, or intolerant, to many of the foods on the lists. Coupled with this, is the likelihood of impaired functional ability, resulting in poor absorption and metabolism of essential nutrients. In this situation, there is no alternative, but to take high daily doses of supplementary nutrients.

One of the more unfortunate effects of nutrient deficiency is referred to by Dr Alexander Schauss, author of *Diet, Crime and Delinquency*.

Insufficient nutrients, toxic metal pollution and food additives are major factors contributing to criminal behaviour. And once an offender is inside, institutional food has been found to aggravate violence and recidivism.

The University of Texas has recently shown that most people need to take daily vitamin and food supplements. According to researchers, a modern diet, providing the necessary daily intake of forty nutrients, would contain 2500 calories. This would be far too fattening for most people and, as such, would be a danger to health. Their conclusions were that, without daily supplements, the modern diet is either undernourishing, or overfattening. This is a very significant finding which should be taken seriously by all people, whether in good health or not. There is also a wealth of evidence to support the fact that urban pollution increases the body's requirement of all nutrients and, here again, the average daily diet, no matter how well contrived, will not provide sufficient quantities to sustain good health.

Many mineral supplements, these days are in chelate form. This process combines minerals, such as zinc, calcium and magnesium, with an amino acid. As a result, better absorption takes place in the intestine, which ensures that the body gets a sufficient amount for its needs. As damage to the upper intestinal tract is so often involved with allergy illness, it is essential that all means possible to improve absorption of nutrients, be employed.

Dr Michael Colgan, in his book, *Your Personal Vitamin Profile*, says that there is never a deficiency of just one vitamin or mineral. Treatment, using only one vitamin or mineral, just does not work. The need is for a complete and balanced blend of all essential nutrients related to each persons biochemical individuality. Lifestyle, age and many other variables, including exposure to pollutants and toxic substances, make up that individuality. Dr Colgan is adamant that the use of nutrients in this way can restore the immune system and provide 'the wonderful continued feeling of well-being, happiness, nobility of mind and the hope of peace.'

There are simple tests available to determine the levels of vitamins and minerals in the body. Minerals are assessed by burning a sample of hair and analysing the ash, using spectro-photometry. Simple blood tests can ascertain vitamin levels. These tests can be carried out by an orthomolecular practitioner.

Orthomolecular nutrient therapy is a major tool in the treatment of allergy illness. It will aid greatly in rebuilding the immune system and reducing food and chemical intolerance. It is best done under the guidance of a qualified practitioner, (not necessarily a medical doctor), however self treatment can also prove beneficial.

Toximolecular drug therapy is often harmful, and contaminates body biochemistry. It is basically the administration of drugs at sub-lethal, or near-lethal, levels. Drugs are alien chemicals which are not normally present in the body's cell structure. They do not halt or prevent disease. At best, they treat symptoms, whilst the underlying disease process continues. Drugs make huge amounts of money for big companies and allow doctors to avoid fuller investigation of symptoms. Multiple allergy sufferers, in particular, will know the complete futility of the toximolecular approach.

Orthomolecular medicine, on the other hand, aims to treat sick cells with the most potent biological weapons possible — nutrients — so that they may rebuild themselves and produce healthy tissues and organs, thus enabling the immune system to function properly once again.

Bio-chemical treatments

Extract from the A.N.Z. M.E. Society newsletter, June 1983 issue

Pam Penman had been ill since the age of six. Her condition fluctuated and, by the time she was in her twenties, her doctors were considering a possible diagnosis of multiple sclerosis. But this proved negative, and more recently a tentative diagnosis of myalgic encephalomyelitis was made. From 1978 on Pam was unable to work and suffered weakness, 'feeling terrible', lack of co-ordination, difficulty in concentration, various aches and pains and nerve twitchings. She was aware of many food allergies, but last November she was hit very hard by almost total sensitivity to her environment, reacting severely to most inhalants. Her weight dropped alarmingly.

Pam and her husband Carl, had read a book *Brain Allergies* by William Philpott, an American doctor specialising in bio-chemical treatments. They contacted him, shortly afterwards mortgaged their home and took off for St Petersburg, Florida. Pam's success story follows:

> Right from the time we first met this incredible man who was bubbling with enthusiasm and always confident of success, we could not help but be encouraged. And with his treatment over a period of eight weeks I grew stronger and stronger, gaining 20 pounds in weight.

Pam was first given a series of treatments involving electrical stimulation of the spine designed to enhance metabolic functioning. She was also tested for most known substances in the body with complex blood and urine analyses (probably not available readily in Australia or New Zealand).

> I was found to be severely deficient in vitamins, minerals, amino acids and enzymes, which had caused an imbalance in my system. Also I underwent thorough food testing and was subsequently placed on a four-day-rotation diet. I was taking numerous nutritional supplements and encouraged to exercise at least thirty minutes per day. These three approaches are maintaining my regained good health. During our stay at the Philpott Medical

Centre we saw many such success stories. From small boys who were autistic or epileptic, to elderly adults who were diabetics or simply had various allergies. They all came with reservations but left feeling there was hope and knowing that within a short time they would be feeling good as new.

Before Pam left for the United States she was indeed horrifically ill. Three months later, she found herself to be 99 per cent well. All symptoms are gone. She no longer reacts to foods or inhalants, but was advised to avoid heavy concentrations of inhalants wherever possible.

16

ENZYMES

The secret of life!

Enzymes control the body's metabolism. Without them, we could not function for a second. Their two main tasks are the digestion of food and the maintenance of tissue and general bodily functions. In simplistic terms, they are similar to a catalyst inasmuch as they enable the release of energy, and the operation of the metabolic processes, to take place at lightning speed. However, whereas catalysts can be used over and over again, enzymes are consumed and must be replaced continuously. An adequate supply of minerals, vitamins and amino acids, from which to make them, is therefore vital to ongoing good health.

Enzymes in digestion

Digestion is the process whereby food is broken down into smaller particles, or molecules, for use in the human body. These digested particles pass through the intestinal wall into the bloodstream, where they are distributed to nourish all parts of the body.

Digestion commences in the mouth, continues in the stomach and duodenum and finalises during the process of chyme (partly digested food) through the small intestine. At each phase of digestion, enzymes are necessary to speed up the various chemical reactions involved. The initial digestive step, that of chewing, is very important. When chewed food is ground into fine particles, the enzymes in the digestive juices can do their work much more effectively. During the chewing action, the food is moistened and mixed with saliva which contains the first of the many different enzymes used throughout the digestive process.

Once the food is swallowed it passes through the esophagus into the stomach, where it is mixed by a vigorous churning motion with more enzyme carrying digestive juices. Protein foods such as meat, eggs and milk commence the digestive process in the stomach, whereas carbohydrates and fats pass through the stomach quickly and commence digestion in the duodenum.

Our eating habits, however, are contrary to this natural process. We tend to eat our carbohydrates and proteins together, and this results in the carbohydrate being held back in the stomach until the protein has been dealt with. The carbohydrate, therefore, stays in the stomach considerably longer than it should which, invariably, leads to fermentation, before it is finally absorbed and eliminated. As a result, continuing stress is placed on the digestive system and a greater production of enzymes is required to digest this fermented material. Also, there is a greater chance of partly undigested food particles passing through the intestinal wall into the bloodstream, where they may cause allergic reactions.

Once the food has passed into the small intestine, the final phase of digestion begins using pancreatic juice, intestinal juice and bile. Pancreatic enzymes, contained in the juice, pour through a duct into the small intestine and mix with intestinal enzymes to finalise digestion. When the food is completely digested it is absorbed by the blood and lymph vessels in the walls of the intestine.

It is easy to see just how vital enzymes are to the maintenance of good health. Unfortunately, the excessive stress, placed on the various enzyme-producing mechanisms of the body by our twentieth century habits, often results in digestion, and assimilation, of food being inefficient for most people. The resultant build-up of toxins leads to widespread illness, such as high blood pressure, arthritis, cancer, heart disease and of course, chronic allergy sickness.

Enzymes are the key to efficient digestion, which in turn leads to a vigorous and healthy life. It is vital that food allergy sufferers appreciate this importance and that they take all possible steps to facilitate efficient use, and production of enzymes in their bodies.

facilitate efficient use, and production of enzymes in their bodies. Awareness of the need to chew food properly, to eat slowly and to eat carbohydrates before proteins, at each meal, can greatly assist a flagging pancreas to recover some of its lost vitality.

Types of enzymes

Salivary

Ptyalin is contained in the saliva and assists in the transformation of some starches to sugar. If food is not chewed properly, adequate amounts of saliva and ptyalin are not produced and digestion immediately gets off to a bad start. This applies particularly to all cereal-derived foods.

Pancreatic

The pancreas waits 'on call' ready to supply a range of digestive enzymes as soon as they are needed. It does not begin to pour its digestive juices into the duodenum until food reaches the intestine. When this happens, two hormones, secretin and pancreozymin, are secreted by the upper small intestine and travel, via the blood, to the pancreas, where they stimulate the secretion of enzyme juice containing a battery of digestive agents. These are:

Trypsin, Chymotrypsin and Carboxypeptidase are the powerful protein-digesting enzymes. If they accumulated in the pancreas they would digest it, so they are secreted in an inactive form, then activated in the intestine. Trypsin and chymotrypsin hydrolyse proteins and polypeptides to peptides whilst caroxypeptidase breaks down the peptides into their component amino acids.

Amylase is similar to ptyalin in function, inasmuch as it converts starches to maltose (malt sugar). Thus, it is responsible for the hydrolysis of carbohydrates and is of particular importance in the digestion of our unhealthy, heavily starch-oriented, diet. Whereas the action of ptyalin is cut short, by acid gastric juice in the stomach, amylase is secreted into the duodenum where it has more leisure to do its work.

Lipase is the fat-digesting enzyme of the pancreas. It converts some fats to monoglycerides and some to glycerol and fatty acids.

Lipases are also secreted by the small intestine, but the pancreatic lipase accounts for about 80 per cent of fat digestion. The emulsifying action of bile prepares the fats for breakdown, by lipase.

Nucleases, Dnase and Rnase are enzymes which break down nucleic acids, from protein foods, into nucleotides, which are compounds that determine gene structure.

Intestinal

Enterokinase — The purpose of this enzyme is to activate the trypsin enzymes from the pancreas. These powerful, protein-digesting enzymes must remain inactive until they reach the intestine, otherwise they would attack the pancreas.

Most of the initial digestive process, in the small intestine, is carried out by enzymes imported from the pancreas. However, contained in the mucosa, covering the intestinal wall, are digestive enzymes which digest food materials whilst they are being absorbed. These enzymes put the finishing touches on the digestion of foodstuffs. In many people, incorrect feeding as an infant, causing intestinal inflammation, has resulted in permanent damage to the intestinal wall and a reduced ability to produce these vital enzymes. In some cases, people have entirely lost the ability to produce one, or several, enzymes, resulting in lifelong allergy to certain foods — milk and cereals being the classical examples.

The enzymes contained in the intestinal mucosa are:

Erepsin which breaks down polypeptides, that are combinations of amino acids found in protein foods, into single amino acids for absorption. Amino acids are regarded as essential to nutrition as they are the building blocks for the proteins which make up most of the body's cells.

Sucrase, Maltase and Lactase — These enzymes further break down, for absorption, sucrose, maltose and lactose, which are the partly digested products of sugars, starches and milk.

It is obvious that without enzymes, we cannot function or without sufficient enzymes we cannot function properly.

Enzyme supplements

People who have impaired enzyme production can gain great benefit from taking enzyme supplements with each meal. This situation could certainly apply to sufferers of food allergy illnesses.

It is possible to obtain several different brands of both pancreatic and intestinal enzymes, however, I would recommend the Bioglan brand as being one of the best available in Australia. This company produces several excellent combinations, in a low allergy base. Allergy sufferers must always be aware that many nutritional supplements contain a yeast base, whilst others have sugars, milk derivatives, wheat starch, artificial additives, etc., which, if taken, will only exacerbate their problems, instead of helping them. The two products most suitable are Active-zyme formula, which contains both pancreatic and intestinal enzymes, and Panazyme 4NF which are pancreatic enzymes.

As has been shown in previous chapters, it is probable that people with food allergy problems have a poor pancreatic output of sodium bicarbonate. Because of this, the pancreatic enzymes are unable to function properly, resulting in partially digested peptides (amino acid combinations), being absorbed into the bloodstream where they induce further allergy reactions. It is important, therefore, to take sodium bicarbonate in conjunction with enzyme supplements. The procedure for taking enzyme supplements is as follows:

1 If enteric-coated, enzymes should be taken before the meal. Products which are not enteric-coated, should be taken towards the end of the meal. If taking Panazyme, or Active-zyme, two tablets should be taken with each meal.

2 Thirty minutes after the meal, two teaspoons of sodium bicarbonate should be taken in a glass of water. This will create an alkaline environment in the duodenum and, thus, allow pancreatic enzymes to function efficiently.

Enzyme levels in life

Dr Edward Howell, in his book, *Food Enzymes for Health and Longevity*, writes:

The fact that the enzyme content of organisms is depleted with increasing old age is forcibly presented when fluids or tissues are examined at different ages. After full mature growth has been attained there is a slow and gradual decrease in the enzyme content of organisms. When the enzyme content becomes so low that metabolism cannot proceed at a proper level, death overtakes the organism.

This decline in enzyme production in the body is due to a variety of reasons, not the least of which is the increasing overload of toxins, caused by a chronic food and chemical allergy condition.

The eating habits of modern mankind further increase toxic overload and speed up the ageing process. The cooking of food is amongst the worst of these habits, and I have found in my own case, that digestion and general health, improved substantially after changing my diet from mainly cooked foods to raw fresh foods. Why is it that cooked foods are so bad for the human body? The answer again is enzymes. Cooked food does not have any enzymes at all! It keeps so well because its natural enzymes, which would otherwise decompose it, have been destroyed. The reason for refrigerated food keeping so well, and frozen food keeping indefinitely, is that enzymes are inhibited by cold. Both cooked food and refrigerated food will only begin to break down when live enzymes are introduced by various microbes in the air. Likewise, preservatives inhibit enzymes, and canned food contains no enzymes.

What does all this mean? It means that, as the bulk of the food we eat contains no enzymes, the body, instead of being able to rely on assistance from natural enzymes in the food, has to produce all the enzymes needed for digestion. This places a continual strain on the digestive system and, as the years go by, results in a declining ability to produce sufficient enzymes for efficient digestion and assimilation of food.

The enzyme content of natural food is proportionate to the amount of calories contained. Fruit is high in enzyme content and is by far, man's most natural and beneficial food. Vegetables contain some enzymes, but not enough to assist the body significantly. When cooked, of course, they contain none. Raw food is the key. Even raw meat and unpasteurised milk contain valuable enzymes, which are lost once cooking, or pasteurisation, takes place. Enzymes contained in raw food, play an important part in relieving the pancreas, and other digestive processes, of extra work. In addition, they are absorbed into the lymph and blood to supplement enzyme production within the body.

Dr Howell's experiments showed that allergenic, partly-digested food particles in the blood, such as yeast, proteins and fats, could be properly digested if there was an adequate level of enzymes present in the blood serum. Thus, they would be removed quickly, instead of remaining to induce allergy responses. Dr Howell was also able to show that, when large doses of enzymes were administered orally, low enzyme levels in the blood returned to normal. It would appear, therefore, that enzyme supplements can be of significant assistance in food allergy illness.

Apart from cooked and processed food, a large proportion of modern diet consists of foods derived from grain products. When you consider breakfast cereals, bread, scones, cakes, biscuits, pie crusts. puddings, sauces, soups, gravy, etc., it makes you realize just how much reliance we place on grains, and their flours, in our everyday diet.

This is a problem because the grains are not easy to digest. Whether they be in wholemeal, or refined form, they pose a big digestive problem for the pancreas. Cereal grains must be cooked before eating because, being a seed, they contain enzyme inhibitors to prevent their destruction. These enzyme inhibitors must be destroyed by cooking, if the human body is to have any chance at all of digesting these foods. Unfortunately, the natural enzymes are also destroyed and, as grains have been constructed by nature to be extremely difficult to break down, the resultant, continual stress on the pancreas over many years of eating these foods, is severe.

Without sufficient enzyme levels, the body cannot function properly and begins to deteriorate. Enzyme levels are high in acute illness, but always low in chronic, or ongoing illness. Food allergy sufferers, invariably, have reduced enzyme levels, due to pancreatic and intestinal dysfunction. It is possible, however, to assist greatly in regaining enzyme efficiency by the following:

Take enzyme supplements daily, followed with bicarbonate of soda.

Eat smaller meals. Much better to have five or six light meals, throughout the day, than three larger ones.

Fast regularly (See Chapter 12)

Take nutritional supplements daily. (See Chapter 15)

Minimise, or avoid entirely, cooked and processed foods.

Do not eat grain products every day.

Do not eat meat every day. Cook as rarely as you can tolerate.

Identify your allergenic foods and avoid them religiously.

Maximise fresh food in your diet, particularly enzyme-rich fruits.

As much as possible, eat single foods at each meal.

ALTERNATIVE MEDICAL STRATEGY

Acupuncture, Shiatsu and Reflexology

Acupuncture is an ancient Chinese method of relieving pain and treating disease, by inserting needles into various parts of the body. This procedure can sometimes be uncomfortable, but has been largely superseded now by painless, electronic acupuncture.

According to Chinese philosophy there are two opposing forces of nature called *Yin* and *Yang*. These are related to the positive and negative energy currents in the body, which are known to exist. When there is a poor balance between *Yin* and *Yang*, disease and pain occurs. Acupuncture improves this balance by changing the flow of energy forces within the body.

Western medicine has not yet been able to explain acupuncture in purely scientific terms. However, a great deal of research, by Western medical scientists, during the past twenty years, has confirmed that it is extremely beneficial in a great number of complex disorders. Acupuncture often succeeds where other medicine fails, and the past few years have seen a great number of European, American and Australian doctors, either specialising in acupuncture, or using it within their general medical practice. German doctors, particularly, have realized the benefits of acupuncture medicine and have been instrumental in developing electronic, diagnostic and treatment methods that are producing excellent results. Dr Reinholdt Voll, in the 1960s, and more recently, Dr Helmut Schimmel are both largely responsible for these developments.

One of the most respected and acclaimed modern physicians in the field of electroacupuncture, is Dr William H. Khoe, of Las Vegas, Nevada. He has been successful in treating people for diseases, which conventional medicine has ignored, (including multiple allergy illness). In recognition of his work, the World Health Organisation has appointed him to its committee on biological medicine. Dr Khoe studied electroacupuncture under the orginator, the great Dr Reinholdt Voll of West Germany. Dr Voll successfully treated himself for terminal cancer, many years ago, using his newly-developed EAV techniques. He has since trained many leading physicians, throughout the world, including Dr Khoe and Dr Kenyon of the United Kingdom. In recognition of his services, Dr Voll has been given a special award by the World Health Organisation, and a medal of honour from the Pope. It is extraordinary that these awards have been made in recognition of his achievements in the advancement of medical practice, yet most general practitioners, through their own ignorance, obstinately refuse to study his teachings, or use his methods. As a consequence, many people, who could otherwise be helped, continue to suffer.

Acupuncture meridians and points

The Chinese believe that there are twelve main meridians, and many more lesser meridians, of energy which connect the body's various organs, both to each other and to a particular part of the body's surface. For instance, the liver is connected to the foot, the stomach to the hand and so on. The meridians are divided into five groups. These are main, connecting, divergent, muscle and extra.

Acupuncture points lie along the lengths of the main meridians. In effect, they are contact points for the organs and link each organ to a particular point on the skin. The Chinese believe that, when the point is stimulated by the insertion of a needle, a profound change in the flow of *chi* (energy) along the meridian, occurs. This, in turn, affects the organ itself. There are 361 named acupuncture points, distributed throughout the body as follows: 75 in the region of the head; 63 on each arm; 139 on the trunk; and 84 are located on each leg. There are also 36 extra points which lie either side of the body, but not along any particular meridian. According to the Peking Academy of Traditional Chinese Medicine, there are, currently, 83 acupuncture points in common use.

One of the most interesting groups of acupuncture points are known as the *Bei-shu* points. They are arranged on the back, at either side of the spine, from the shoulder blades downwards. These points are linked to the lung, heart, liver, stomach, kidney, large and small intestines and bladder. Discovering the precise location of a tender area of the back, enables the acupuncturist to diagnose which organ is diseased. Stimulating a *Bei-shu* point is believed to assist the damaged organ to regain function. As discussed in Chapter 7, food and chemical allergies can damage the major organs of the body by the accumulation of toxins. Allergy sufferers often do experience positive results from acupuncture, especially once the allergens are identified and avoided.

Benefits to allergy sufferers

In addition to stimulating organs to regain function, acupuncture has also been found useful in the direct control of pain, and other symptoms, arising from allergy illness. Whilst care must be taken to ensure that relief of the symptom, or symptoms, does not distract focus from the underlying cause, acupuncture treatment can, nevertheless, be an effective palliative. Common allergy symptoms such as back pains, asthma, respiratory infections, constipation, eczema, limb pains, headaches, hypertension, catarrh and tinnitus are examples of symptoms that can be relieved, or reduced, by the regular application of acupuncture.

The major benefit to be derived, as mentioned earlier, is the toning-up effect that acupuncture can have on the major organs. After years of labouring in an overloaded, toxic body, the major organs, particularly the pancreas, liver, kidneys and intestine, become weakened and suffer impaired function. In conjunction with dietary control, acupuncture can be extremely beneficial in stimulating these organs to commence the recovery process.

In my own case, Dr Kenyon selected the acupuncture points of liver three, stomach thirty-six, liver eleven and triple warmer ten. On my arrival back in Australia, I consulted an acupuncturist (who is also a medical doctor) and underwent an initial course of ten weekly treatments, followed by a booster every few weeks. I have since had further weekly treatments intermittently. The beneficial effect of these treatments over a period of time, has been significant, and I recommend all allergy sufferers to consult a qualified acupuncturists as part of their plan to overcome their illness, and recover their zest for living.

It is necessary, and important, to persevere with acupuncture over a period of time. Some extremely sensitive people such as myself, may appear initially to suffer adverse reactions. These may show in the form of fatigue, dizziness and, perhaps, nausea after the first few treatments. Do not be alarmed. Wait in the acupuncturist's office until the symptoms have disappeared, and then go home to rest. Rest is important after an acupuncture treatment if you are to receive maximum benefit. Reactions, such as these, are positive and indicate that organs are being goaded into action by the stimulation process. You will find after a few visits, that these after-effects will disappear and will be replaced by a sense of well being, which can often last for some time.

It must be clear, however, that acupuncture is not, in itself, a cure. It is a valuable aid in the rebuilding of the immune system, and the recovery of one's general health. It is part of the multi-faceted approach necessary to overcome a multiple allergy condition successfully. Prime consideration, of course, must always be given to identifying the offending allergens and removing them from diet and environment.

How acupuncture works

Although it has not yet been conclusively proven, there is a great weight of evidence to suggest that acupuncture relates to the autonomic nervous system. This is the part of the nervous system which controls involuntary reactions, such as breathing and digestion, and involves the continuous function of all major organs.

Dr James Reilly, who was Director of the Claude Bernard Hospital Laboratory in Paris, for over forty years, discovered that mild stimulation of the nervous system, by electrical means, was of great benefit in assisting the body to reject disease. He found that the nervous system, under conditions of disease and illness, needed to be 'diverted' from its tendency to aggravate a diseased condition. Once this happened, the pressure on the immune system was eased and the body began to recover.

It is conceivable that the needle effect of acupuncture may work in a similar way. The Chinese claim that the body's immune system can be modified by acupuncture. In the treatment of malaria, for instance, in Chinese hospitals, needles are inserted a short time before the expected rigors. Following acupuncture, the rigors do not appear, and the malaria parasites disappear from the blood.

Acupuncture works, there is no doubt about that, to what degree depends upon the individual and the nature of the illness. It is highly recommended to all those suffering from allergy illness, to be used as a useful tool, rather than a panacea.

Therapeutic massage — Shiatsu

Therapeutic massage, like acupuncture, originated from the Chinese. Over the centuries it travelled through the Korean Peninsula to Japan where it has undergone extensive refinement. Today, it has reached the stage where it is surprisingly effective in obtaining relief for many ailments.

Shiatsu is gaining in popularity in Western countries, as part of the move away from the drug-taking and pill-popping of conventional medicine as we know it. Instead of the dangerous and often crude approach of interfering with the body's chemical system, by the use of potent drugs (from which there are often poisonous side-effects), the body is stimulated to produce its own healing. In other words, Shiatsu, like acupuncture, stimulates positive chemical reactions in the body, to commence the healing process.

Although termed massage, Shiatsu is really a very specific and regimented therapy, based on principles which are as complex as, and similar to, acupuncture. It involves massage and pressure being applied to specific parts of the body to relieve symptoms and to assist in the regeneration of diseased organs. Shiatsu makes use of the principle that organic disorders have surface manifestations. Among the nervous reflex systems of the body, one of the most representative is the mechanism whereby organic disorders give out symptoms which affect skin and muscles. The surface, and near-surface parts of the body constantly receive stimuli from the brain and spinal cord, by way of the network of nerves that extends over the entire body. When one of the inner organs is out of order, a corresponding stiffness, or soreness, will occur in the skin and muscles. In addition, dry scaly patches of skin are further signs of the autonomic nervous system indicating organic disorder.

How Shiatsu works

As internal abnormalities exert an influence on the surface of the body, it follows that internal organs can be influenced by means of stimuli on the body's surface. For example, by applying pressure to a part of the body's surface, it is possible to stimulate the spinal cord and other nerves of the central nervous system. It has been proven scientifically that such stimulus activates internal organs, is beneficial to blood vessels and produces chemical changes, such as the secretion of vital hormones. In other words, organic disorders can be helped by stimulus, in the form of rubbing and exerting pressure to the appropriate spot, or position, on the body.

Shiatsu treatment

A general form of treatment for allergies, relates to the localised, or generalised, itching, rash or swelling which invariably accompanies allergy reactions. These may pass in a matter of days, or weeks, or they may be chronic and persist for months, or years.

According to Professor Katsusuke Serizewa, of Tokyo University, people with allergies frequently have rashes or dry, scaly areas on the back, in a triangular area, running from the base of the neck to the outer edges of the shoulder blades. In addition to this, if pressure is applied with the thumb to the seventh cervical vertebra — located level with the top of the shoulders — it will produce a sudden, sharp pain. Repeated massage at this point will greatly assist in reducing allergy symptoms. To extend the benefits of this treatment further, it should be followed by massage and gentle pressure at the following points: either side of the third and ninth thoracic vertebrae; either side of the second and fourth lumbar vertebrae; centre of the chest; centre of the diaphragm; below the navel, and the outside centre of each wrist.

Shiatsu can be of great benefit to allergy sufferers. However, like acupuncture, it should be used in conjunction with the other methods suggested in this book, and not in itself as a means of cure. The advantage of Shiatsu is that it can be safely carried out by practically anybody, once they know the points at which to apply pressure.

Reflexology

The principles of reflexology are similar to those of both acupuncture and Shiatsu, inasmuch as all three are based on the principle that internal disorders can be corrected by external stimulation. Reflexology differs from the others in that it involves only the feet or hands.

It has been confirmed, by scientific tests in recent years, that internal disorders do, indeed, manifest themselves on the body surfaces in the form of lumps, rashes and muscular tenderness. These symptoms are not, necessarily, located immediately adjacent to the malfunctioning organ, and it seems, in a great number of cases, the reverse is true.

Reflexologists look mainly to the feet for both diagnosis and treatment, and have long since come to associate certain areas of the foot (mainly on the sole) with specific organs. Hence, if the small intestine is in trouble it reflects in soreness in the arch region of the sole, or, if the lungs are a problem, the top of the foot immediately above the toes will be tender, and so on. By therapeutic massage and pressure, applied to the tender area, a corresponding beneficial effect will be conveyed to the damaged organ. Here again, it seems that the autonomic nervous system is stimulated to cease 'attacking' the organ, or bodily system, at fault, thus making it easier for the body to operate its own healing mechanisms effectively.

Any form of natural healing method, which is designed to assist the body's own healing mechanism, must be of benefit to allergy sufferers. Remember, an ongoing allergy condition can damage the cells and internal organs, causing further allergies and other illness. The resultant clogging of both blood and lymph systems with toxic matter, places the major organs under continual stress and causes them to start wearing out.

Reflexology has been found to be of particular benefit to the lymphatic system, the kidneys, the liver, and the digestive system. It is probably complementary to acupuncture, and may be considered as an additional source of assistance to allergy sufferers, during a planned recovery programme.

COLONIC HEALTH

A vital aid to recovery

One of the inevitable side effects of food allergy illness is constipation. Invariably, allergy sufferers will experience recurring trouble with this insidious allergy symptom, throughout their lives. Attempts to rectify the problem will always fail, until the allergenic food is detected and removed from the diet.

Dr Vayda, in his book, *Health for Life*, says that, due to modern medical care, more and more babies are surviving with errors of metabolism, suspect enzyme and other genetic deficiencies, which make digestion of some foods difficult for them. As discussed in earlier chapters, grains are notoriously difficult to digest and pose great strain on an imperfect digestive system.

However, it is not only cereal foods that are a problem. Studies have shown that the intestine can be partially 'paralysed' by a large influx of any allergenic matter, causing a marked slowing down in the digestive and evacuative processes. Chronic constipation, therefore, can be regarded as one of the major signs, and major symptoms, of an unrecognized food allergy condition. Unfortunately, when this problem has been going on for years, as often is the case, damage may result to the colon. When this happens, doctors diagnose diverticulitis, colitis, cancer, or some other colonic disease, as the cause. Whereas, what they should be looking at is what caused the 'cause'. Often, the original problem will be a continuing reaction, by the body, to an allergenic food, or foods, eaten unwittingly over many years. Remember, that to an allergic person, allergenic food is toxic and what he is doing by eating it, is slowly poisoning himself — possibly to death.

Mention was made in Chapter 7 of the effects of allergies on the body and the term 'target organ' was used. Not only can the colon, itself, become a target organ, as the result of slow processing of fermenting, toxin-laden rubbish, but the liver, also, can be affected. The colon completes the digestive process by mulching the chyme and absorbing the remaining liquids and nutrients into the bloodstream, which are then returned to the liver for processing. Toxin-laden allergenic matter, entering the bloodstream, can cause further problems by prolonging allergic reactions and overloading the liver. As a result, the liver ceases to do its work effectively, and this leads to further toxic overload in the body.

Therefore, keeping the colon free of slow-moving allergenic matter is of vital importance. Whilst this material is still in your body, you will continue to suffer from allergy symptoms. Once it is evacuated, or removed, your symptoms will begin to disappear, providing you avoid intake of further allergenic substances.

Keeping the colon clean, achieves two purposes. Firstly, it will prevent the deterioration of the colon itself into a spastic and, finally, diseased state. Secondly, it will ensure that symptoms are minimised by shortening the time that allergenic matter remains in the body. Obviously, the best way of helping the colon is to avoid allergenic foods, but this is often not a simple process, taking time, perhaps many months, before the individual's allergens are fully identified. Even after this has happened, it may be that he, or she, will choose to eat allergenic food, from time to time, simply to provide a dietary change, or because there is nothing else available. If this is done occasionally, it should not cause undue harm, however while this food remains in the body, allergic reactions and temporary damage will take place. Dr N.W. Walker, a world renowned authority on the colon, says in his book, *Colon Health, The Key to a Vibrant Life* (published by Norwalk Press)

the elimination of undigested food and other waste products is equally as important as the proper digestion and assimilation of food. In fact, because of the danger of the inevitable effects of toxaemia, of toxic poisons, as the outcome of the neglected accumulation and failure to expel faeces, debris and other waste matter from the body, I can think of nothing more significant or vital! Few of us realize that failure to effectively eliminate waste products from the body causes so much fermentation and putrefaction in the larger intestine, or colon, that the neglected accumulation of such waste can, and frequently does, result in a lingering demise.

Constipation

The word 'constipation' comes from the Latin word *constipatus* which means 'to cram' or 'pack together'. The packed accumulation of faeces in the bowel makes evacuation difficult. This can come about because of the semi-paralytic effect of allergenic matter on the intestine. The resultant slowing down of bowel movement results in a clogging effect, leading to constipation.

A state of constipation may also exist when bowel movements seem to be normal. This is due to allergenic food leaving a coating of slime on the inner walls of the colon, like plaster. As time progresses, this coating will increase in thickness until there is only a narrow tube, through which the faeces can pass for final evacuation. This causes a back-up of faeces in pockets within the colon, resulting in distortion of the colon, malfunction and disease. It will also affect the final digestive process, resulting in the passage of undigested food, from which the body derives little, or no benefit.

The coating, or faecal incrustation on the inside of the colon, partially or totally, prevents the infusion of the intestinal flora necessary for colon lubrication. These normally come from glands in the walls of the first half of the colon. As a result, not only is the passage of faeces restricted by the narrowing aperture, but, also, by the lack of lubrication, resulting in a 'sticky' contact with the colon walls. This results in a gradual build-up of the coating, which, increasingly, blocks the bowel and becomes a continuing generator of toxicity. Not a happy picture!

Use of laxatives to rectify constipation is safe enough, occasionally. However, when the bowel has become impacted to the point where constant use is necessary, it becomes a very dangerous situation indeed. Many people do not realize that laxatives work by irritating the bowel. This causes it to go into a paroxysm of movement in order to expel the laxative, and anything loose in the bowel goes with it. It has been found that the use of laxatives and cathartics are not only habit forming, but decidedly destructive to the membrane of the intestines. They disturb the natural rhythm of the excretory organs, which demand increasingly heavier doses until the point of no return is reached. Permanent damage may, eventually, require a colostomy. It is not necessary for this to happen, as in many cases, a series of colonic irrigations can remove impacted, allergenic material and help restore normal bowel function.

Colonic irrigation

A colonic irrigation is, in effect, a glorified enema, using, perhaps, a hundred, to a hundred and twenty, litres of water during a half hour, to one hour, period. The patient lies relaxed on an appropriate table and is connected to the colonic equipment, by a trained operator, who controls water flow and explusion, throughout the treatment.

It is a painless, and efficient, procedure to remove accumulated faecal matter from the bowel. It is of particular value, in that it can reach along the full length of the colon to the cecum — something which the enema cannot do. Thus, the vital digestive and peristaltic processes, of the first half of the colon, can be improved and, eventually, returned to normality by a number of treatments. This number may vary from six to twenty, or more depending on the degree of compactment. The colonic process allows the plaster-like coating to be thoroughly soaked and saturated with plain water. This enables its removal gradually, and comfortably, without causing the inner lining of the colon to become raw and painful.

Modern colonic equipment incorporates the injection of oxygen into the colon, together with the water. This process was invented back in 1938 by Dr Roy W. De Welles who, for years, was considered to be the outstanding authority in America, on diseases of the colon and methods for their recovery. European investigators, at the time, reported the results of tests of this treatment. They found that pint doses of oxygen, injected into the body by way of colonic irrigation, were more beneficial than hundreds of gallons taken by inhalation. The most dramatic results came from the application of oxygen to bowel disorders. Because putrefactive bacteria, abounding in these conditions, are anaerobic, they cannot live in the presence of oxygen. Consequently when oxygen is introduced, these germs are rapidly destroyed and normality can return.

Apart from the flushing and cleansing effect of the water, it also has a therapeutic effect on the intricate system of nerves and blood vessels within the colon. Proper regulation of water temperatures, by the operator, results in increased blood supply to the colon, greatly assisting in normalising its function.

It is important to realize that there are practically no sensory (pain-recording) nerves in the colon. This explains why people can often develop colonic disease, to a terminal state, before they are aware of any trouble. Thus, an allergy-caused pollution in the bloodstream can be developing without the victim being any the wiser, except that he feels bad and does not know why. The resultant poisons, generated in the lower bowel, will attack tissues, organs and glands which are congenitally the weakest. The result may be impairment of the kidneys, Bright's disease, damage to the pancreas, diabetes, stomach ulcers, high blood pressure, cancer and so on. Therefore, the ramifications of allowing allergenic matter to impact and ferment in the bowel, year after year become obvious. There is only one result — serious illness, followed by major surgery, and even death.

It has been shown, over many years, that some serious conditions of the colon can be reversed and, eventually, cured by colonic irrigation. For allergy sufferers, not only is there an immediate benefit, that of removing allergens from the body, but also a longer term benefit — that of ensuring that accumulating toxins from an impacted colon, do not continue circulating in the body, to cause further disease and eventual death.

Colonic irrigation is relatively inexpensive, painless and effective. Many food allergy sufferers will have a degree of malfunction of the colon, due to impacted allergenic matter. Therefore, as part of the recovery process, allergy sufferers should consider colonic irrigation as one of the options that can help a return to efficient bowel function. If you decide to undergo colonic irrigation, ensure that it is carried out under medical supervision, by properly trained operators. Within these guidelines, I have found the procedure to be safe and effective. However, if you have any doubts, you should consult your doctor.

The enema

Whereas a colonic irrigation is carried out by a trained operator, using special equipment, an enema is a simple exercise which can be carried out regularly at home. It involves an enema bag, a piece of rubber tubing and an anal syringe, or nozzle. The difference between a colonic irrigation and an enema is that, whereas the colonic irrigation will penetrate the full length of the colon to its beginning (the cecum), the enema will only reach some of the way. Therefore, the vital first half, where final absorption of nutrients takes place, is not benefited. Impaction may still occur along this section.

However, if the lower part of the colon, that is, the descending colon, sigmoid and rectum, are cleansed, when necessary, with an enema, the ascending and transverse colon will also benefit, indirectly. This is because a clean lower colon will hasten the passage of faeces from the upper colon, thus reducing opportunity for impaction and fermentation.

Food allergy sufferers often have an irritated bowel, whether they realize it or not. A regular enema can be extremely helpful in reducing irritation and removing sluggish, fermenting, allergenic matter. This helps to reduce symptoms and to free the system of overloading toxins.

The enema is a simple and extremely useful aid for allergy sufferers. Particularly because it costs nothing and can be done in the comfort and privacy of one's own home. However, care should be taken to ensure that it is not done too often, so as to become habit forming.

It has been shown in this chapter that continuous ingestion of allergenic food can lead to chronic bowel problems, of which the victim may be semi-ignorant. The result is further toxic overload and likelihood of organic disease. A few years ago, at the Royal

Society of Medicine, London, Dr William Hunter, talking on alimentary toxaemia, said:

> The fact that chronic constipation might exist in certain individuals as an almost permanent condition, without apparently causing ill health, is due solely to the power and protective action of the liver. It is not evidence of the comparative harmlessness of constipation per se, but only an evidence that some individuals possess the cecum and the colon of an ox, with the liver of a pig, capable of doing any amount of detoxification.

Some 'fortunate' individuals can, indeed, abuse their bodies and get away with it for a long time. Others can't. Often, the cumulative effects of food allergy can result in auto-intoxication from an inflamed and impacted bowel. Internal cleansing, with colonic irrigation and enemas, can be a useful part of the multi-faceted approach, needed to overcome food and chemical allergy illness.

EXERCISE

Know how to use it

I want to take this opportunity to thank you for the aerobics conditioning programme. I have followed this programme faithfully for over nine months. During the past six months, I have been averaging as least thirty points per week entirely by walking. I sleep better, feel better and have gone through the winter without any medical problems for the first time in years—and I am anxiously awaiting my ninety-fourth year.

The above is an extract from a letter published in Dr Kenneth H. Cooper's, now famous book, *The New Aerobics*. This book has probably been more responsible than any other for educating people world-wide to the fact that aerobic exercise is probably the best form of exercise for the maintenance of good health.

It must be emphasised that exercise alone will not achieve, or maintain, good health. There has been a universally popular misconception for years, that exercise will protect the body against all forms of dietary abuse. This is simply not so. Without careful attention to diet, regular exercise will do no more than slow down the inevitable downward slide to chronic illness and degenerative disease. However, regular exercise is that other essential ingredient, which, together with the right dietary approach, will ensure the maintenance of vigor and robustness well into old age.

Types of exercise

There are basically four different types of exercise. These are:

1 **Isometrics**—This involves the contracting of muscles, with a minimum of movement. It is useful to prevent wasting of muscles but does not contribute to overall health.

2 **Isotonics**—These include exercises such as callisthenics and weight lifting. Although these exercises involve more stretching and contracting than isometrics, little oxygen is used. The resultant increase in strength and suppleness, therefore, will not, necessarily, do much to enhance good health. It can, however, tend to reduce the effect of bad health habits.

3 **Anaerobics**—There is more movement in this form of exercise than either isometrics or isotonics. However, the additional need for oxygen is still fairly minimal. Anaerobic exercise include short walks and brief sprints. They are not prolonged enough to produce a 'training effect'.

4 **Aerobics**—This is a system of exercise which relates oxygen consumption to physical fitness. It is designed to promote the supply, and use, of oxygen by the body. It involves continuous exercise which demands oxygen, but not to a greater extent than the lungs can provide. Progressive training will increase oxygen capacity and improve health.

Allergies and aerobics

While a careful programme of identification and avoidance of allergenic foods and chemicals will set the sufferer on the road to recovery, there is no greater way of speeding up that process than by the careful, regular use of aerobic exercise. Initially, some walking, gradually increasing in distance and duration, is the correct method. In time, some running can be alternated with walking and, finally, regular, relaxed running, or jogging, will achieve better health in a shorter time.

Unless there are mechanical or locomotive reasons why you cannot do aerobic exercise, then you are wasting your time doing anything else. Age is no barrier. Nathan Pritikin, at the Pritikin

Research Foundation, California, found that a combination of diet, and carefully staged aerobic exercise, dramatically improved the most extreme cases of degenerative illnesses, such as arthritis, atherosclerosis, arteriosclerosis and heart disease. Researchers at the Pritikin Foundation, have found that the body actually rejuvenates itself, if given the right type of exercise, coupled with a clean, low allergenic diet. A tremendous, living example of this research is personified by Mrs Eula Weaver of California. At eighty-one, she was crippled with heart disease and arthritis, and could not walk more than 30 metres. Her 'days' were, literally, numbered. Introduced to the Pritikin diet and an aerobic exercise programme, she began to improve. After four years, at eighty-five, she won a gold medal, at the Senior Olympics, in both the half mile and mile events. The following year, she picked up two more golds. Now aged ninety-one, she can still run a mile every day.

Leading allergists, worldwide, are in agreement about two things. Firstly, food and chemical intolerance is a major cause of degenerative illness. Secondly, regular aerobic exercise is essential in the recovery process. It is important, however, to keep your exercise programme well within your physical capabilities at that time. As Dr Cooper says:

> One basic rule to be aware of in entering an exercise programme is this: Avoid straining and pushing yourself to the extent that you become over fatigued. Such intense effort at the outset of an exercise programme is not only dangerous, it also defeats your basic purpose. Instead of feeling more fit and vigorous, you'll just feel chronically tired.

For those who have been severly affected by food and chemical intolerances for quite some time, beware! Your body will have been considerably hammered, and your ability to recover from exercise greatly impaired. The initial emphasis must be on extreme caution. Ensure that your exercise programme does not fully utilise your existing capacity. Any attempt to ignore this principle, and to rush into a strenuous exercise programme, will be counter productive, to the point where, no matter how clean your diet is, all the old symptoms will flare up in triplicate. Your body needs time to adjust. A very gradual process will help the body recover its full biochemical function and, at the same time, leave you with a steadily increasing feeling of well-being.

Dr R. W. Gorringe, a New Zealand expert, speaking on multiple allergy illness, found that,

> There are some other parts that it is important to know about, in terms of the programme for recovery. One involves the use of aerobic exercise. This is exercise done at a quarter effort—whether it is skipping, jogging on the spot at home, jogging rebounder, trampoline, swimming, or riding a bicycle. You go at such a level that you puff and pant but at a level that you think you could go on and on. Start with three minutes a day, i.e. that level, where if you stopped, by five or six breaths you could be back to normal. It appears that if people will exercise at that level, starting at a very small level and building up from there, there are many of the oxygenase enzymes in the body that are currently inoperative, that will then be turned on again.

Effects of regular exercise

Some ongoing benefits from regular exercise are:

Red cells   These may undergo a permanent increase by as much as 30 per cent.

White cells — It is known that a vigorous increase takes place with some permanent effect. Lymphocytes can increase, permanently, by up to 60 per cent. (These are the cells from which both red and white blood cells are renewed.)

Lactic Acid — Increased lung capacity, through regular training, makes the expulsion of lactic acid far more effective. Lactic acid is broken down into carbon dioxide and water, which is then expelled by the lungs, with greater efficiency, as fitness increases.

Oxygen — The tissues absorb about twice as much oxygen, during vigorous exercise, as when the body is at rest. Because of other factors, such as widening of the capillaries and the fact that the heart pumps up to five times more blood during exercise, the total oxygen supply can increase to about twenty times the rest value. This process helps cleanse and rejuvenate the body.

Cholesterol—Exercise has a beneficial effect on cholesterol levels in the blood. One study in Finland, found that 'the serum-cholesterol content in long-distance skiers' men as well as women, is clearly lower than that of the average person and that the content is no higher in older skiers than in the younger ones, although in the population as a whole the cholesterol content increases with age.'

Rheumatism and arthritis—In recent years, many studies have found that regular exercise significantly contributes to the prevention of these diseases.

Ageing — The value of regular, physical exercise can be clearly seen in studies done during a gymnastic and athletic festival, held at Marburg, Germany. Participants were men, aged forty to eighty-four years, and women, aged thirty to fifty-two. Analysis of results showed that, as a group, the participants in regular training were, physiologically, at least ten years younger than ordinary people of the same biological age. Other research has shown that the time for the appearance of degenerative disease of old age can be delayed by regular physical exercise.

Heart—People who exercise regularly, often have pulse rates of 60, or lower, at rest. (The average rate is around 72 for non-exercisers.) Recent research has shown that the lower the heart rate, the less chance of heart disease. A well-conditioned heart develops extra capillaries, which increase collateral circulation. Increased collateral circulation has been shown to be a major factor in the prevention, or avoidance, of heart attacks.

Enzymes—Enzyme activity increases in the body, and oxygenase enzymes, which may have been largely inactive for years, become reactivated. The general toning-up effect on the pancreas and intestine, due to increased supplies of richer, better oxygenated blood, will result in these organs producing more enzymes.

Detoxification—This process is considerably enhanced, owing to the major organs being fed greater quantities of better blood and due to the resultant increase in flow, along with a corresponding stimulation to the lymph system and the endocrine system. Also, metabolism and absorption improve as a result of regular aerobic exercise. It is important, however, not to exceed stress limitations, as this can result in an overload of lactic acid and cause further symptoms.

Lactic acid

One of the by-products of physical exercise is lactic acid. This comes about because exercise causes a breakdown of stored sugar, to produce energy. Lactic acid is a residue from this process and can remain in the body in an ionic form known as lactate. Allergy sufferers tend to accumulate higher levels of lactic acid than healthy people, due to the extra stress placed on their bodies by the illness.

It is interesting to note that lactic acid is the common organic acid, found in milk and other dairy products that have turned sour. It also occurs in sauerkraut, pickles and beer, three well-known allergy-causing foods.

Lactic acid has a tendency to 'tie up' circulating calcium, thus making it unavailable for the body's normal metabolic requirements. Calcium supplements are, therefore, essential during any ongoing exercise programme. Firstly, to neutralise the imflammatory effects of too much lactic acid in blood, muscles and tissues, and secondly, to ensure that the body has an adequate supply of vital calcium, for its other requirements. Essentially, calcium should always be taken together with magnesium and in similar dosages. Vitamin D is also essential for proper calcium absorption, and one excellent source of this vitamin, if you are tolerant to it, is cod liver oil.

Lactic acid inflammation is a problem for anyone who is unfit and commencing an exercise programme. Therefore it is important to build up slowly, so that the body can develop the capacity to deal with it effectively.

Types of aerobic exercise

The most functional of aerobic exercises are walking, running (including jogging) swimming and cycling. At the start of an exercise programme, the best form of exercise is walking. This can begin with five minutes a day, or even less—whatever is well within your capacity. The important thing is to build up slowly, so that you do not incur either mental, or physical stress, which your depleted state of health cannot handle. Possibily, more exercise programmes have been aborted, due to initial impatience and overexertion, than for any other reason.

After a gradual build-up of your walking program, over six to eight weeks, you can increase the pace, if you want to, by changing to running or cycling, still taking care to stay well within your relative physical capacity. However, there is no need to change. If you are happy with your walking programme, and making progress, then stay on it. As a rough rule of thumb, a 30 minute walk, covering 3 km daily, with no after-affects, would mean that you had regained a reasonable standard of health and fitness. Alternatively, if you are running, then 15 minutes per day, covering 3 km, will equate to 30 minutes of walking. These guidelines are based on exercising five days per week.

It is important that any exercise programme should incorporate a gradual build-up over a period of time. A recent publication, entitled *You and Stress* suggests that an eight week programme, initially, should be aimed at building up muscle tissue. This is because the muscles, and blood vessels supplying them have actually shrunk and have to be rebuilt to provide the extra capacity needed. It suggests a daily ten minute exercise plan as follows:

1 Exercise to stretch the muscles for one minute.

2 Exercises which push muscles to maximum effort (such as push-ups or weight lifting) for four minutes.

3 Exercises that create endurance (such as skipping and jogging) for five minutes.

Although this programme is a good guide, it is important to remember that intensity is not all that important. People with toxic overload, from foods and chemicals, should take care to work well within their current capacity, otherwise the exercise will overstress an already tired body. In a recent study at the University of Colorado, it was found that the amount of time spent on the exercise, was more important than the intensity of the exercise, for a range of benefits, including reduction in cholesterol levels. Although they found diet and exercise to be the best ways to reduce cholesterol, it did not reduce faster if the exercise was intensified. Therefore, regular, rhythmic exercise seems to be more important to improve health than intense, vigorous effort.

Although walking, running and cycling are excellent, aerobic exercises, and are all that is required to increase aerobic capacity, a possible drawback is that they are, basically, leg exercises. It is not essential to exercise the upper body to produce an adequate training effect. However, those who require good muscle tone in the arms and chest, should also consider either swimming, or callisthenics, twice per week. Care must be taken to avoid overstressing the body, and it may be necessary to reduce the duration of aerobic training on those days.

If your weight is normal, you are avoiding allergens and you have begun exercising regularly, you should be well on the road to recovery from, or control of, a food/chemical allergy problem. Within a short time, you should be sleeping better and feeling more energetic. Don't be surprised if you find you need less sleep. Often, physical fitness produces more energy and more time to enjoy it, due to the quality of sleep being vastly improved. If you find that you are having trouble sleeping, it will probably mean that you are exercising beyond your current capacity, so cut back, to avoid overstress.

An example of a low, allergenic diet, combined with plenty of aerobic exercise is described by Dr J. W. Postma, in his book, *Physical Education,* in which he says:

A study of peoples like the Hunzas, a small nation of 30,000 souls who live in the Himalaya Mountains in Asia, is very instructive for the study of the part physical movement plays in the maintenance of fitness. Besides a diet of fruit, vegetables and beans, (only 20 per cent of the food is cooked) and particularly of apricots and oil from apricot pips, sport (swimming in ice cold water, climbing and hunting) plays an important part in keeping the nation fit. Many people reach the age of 100; diseases like cancer, tuberculosis and measles are unknown, and there are no heart attacks or cases of high blood pressure. This example of the simple way of life, plenty of movement in the open air, little smoking and a healthy diet is worth following.

To summarise the advantages of regular exercise, I could not fault a paragraph from the *Nutrition Almanac*:

A healthy body is the result of proper nutrition combined with a regular pattern of physical exercise. Exercise imparts vigor and activity to all organs and secures and maintains healthy integrity of all their functions. Exercise improves the tone and quality of muscle tissue and stimulates the processes of digestion, absorption, metabolism and elimination. It also strengthens blood vessels, lungs and heart, resulting in improved transfer of oxygen to the cells and increased circulation of the blood and lymph systems. Exercise develops grace, poise and symmetry of the body, helps in correcting defective development or injuries and stimulates the mind.

What more is there to say!

A careful programme of aerobic exercise, always well within capacity, together with avoidance of allergens, is an essential factor in the recovery process to sustain good health.

STRESS

You can control it

It is a fact that, irrespective of cause, an overdose of stress will often provoke yearnings for allergenic substances, which will ultimately create more stress. This vicious cycle must be avoided at all costs.

Much has been written about stress in some highly specialised books on the subject. Dr Hans Selye, in his books *Stress of Life* and *Stress without Distress*, has opened the way to a whole new understanding of the effects of stress, both internal and external, on the psychological and physiological workings of the body.

Stress is an essential part of life. It is always present, in varying degrees, and it is impossible to avoid completely. What is possible however, is the management and control of stress, so that it has a productive, rather than counter-productive, effect on the biological and sociological life of the individual. In *Stress of Life*, Dr Selye explains that, although stress can be destructive, it can also be enjoyable. Without stress, we could not enjoy the great triumph of winning a race, the joy of having a baby or the satisfaction of passing examination finals. Stress, at times, is a great motivator, but it is necessary to monitor our daily exposure to stress to ensure that our bodies are not being overburdened. An overload of stress is like an overload of toxins, with the destructive effect on the body's biochemistry being virtually identical.

Effect on the body

Dr Selye defines stress as 'the non-specific response of the body to any demand made upon it.' By 'non-specific' he means responses which are not visable or obvious.

When the body is placed under stress the endocrine system is affected. As previously discussed, the endocrine system comprises the pineal, pituitary, thyroid, thymus, pancreas, adrenals, ovaries and testes. Of particular interest to allergy sufferers is the pancreas. This gland is probably more primarily affected than any other part of the body, by the stress of ongoing food and chemical intolerances. However, when the body is placed under stress from other sources, for example, an external threat to one's physical safety, the adrenal glands trigger off a flash of biochemical reaction which involves all the other endocrine glands.

In particular, the adrenal glands release glucocorticoids, to increase blood sugar and so provide the extra energy needed to deal with the emergency. When the excitement is over, the pancreas is supposed to secrete extra insulin, to bring the blood sugar back to normal. If the pancreas is affected by allergy illness, it may already be overworked and oversensitive to changes in blood sugar. As it has been seen with ongoing food allergy problems, particularly refined carbohydrate addiction, the pancreas, through overwork and hypertrophy overreacts when confronted with increased sugar levels and produces too much insulin. The result is a lowering of blood sugar to below the normal levels, with the resultant fatigue, depression, aching and other symptoms of hypoglycaemia. In other words, external stress is bad news for allergy sufferers as it places further load on a system which is already exhausted, by the continuing internal stress of food and chemical intolerances.

In addition, an external crisis results in cortisone being secreted by the adrenals to dampen down the body's immune responses. This is to allow the body to operate at maximum efficiency, often in spite of quite serious injury, in order that escape from a threatening or harmful situation, can take place. If the body is placed under stress constantly, or if cortisone is administered in drug form too frequently, the immune system becomes used to being 'dampened down' and ceases to function efficiently. In this condition, the thymus gland, which controls the body's immune system, becomes shrunken and ineffectual. The lymphocytes (white cells), which defend the body against antigens and other invaders, cease to function effectively. The resultant high viscosity of the blood, and sluggish flow, causes poor oxygen delivery to the tissues. The whole scene is set for a relentless deterioration in health. This is bad news for the allergy sufferer, as he is already in trouble with a malfunctioning immune system. Additional stress, therefore, will compound this problem.

According to Dr John Jemmot, of Princeton University, stress makes you more susceptible to allergies and infections. Research carried out at the University, showed that stress reduces the production of IgA immunoglobulin, thereby reducing the capacity of the immune system to deal effectively, with food and chemical antigens. IgA forms a protective coating on the body's mucosa surfaces, such as in the nasal passages and the intestine. Reduced production in the intestine can, amongst other things, lead to increased food/chemical intolerance. Reduced IgA in the nasal passages will contribute to intolerance of inhaled substances.

External stress need not be physical. In this modern life of ours it is more likely to be caused by one of the many problems encountered while just getting through the day. Such things as a crisis in the office, driving to work in heavy traffic, marital problems, and examinations: all are common examples of external factors placing stress on the body. These factors, although phsychological in origin, are just as valid, and equally devastating to body biochemistry, as the biochemical havoc caused by food and chemical allergies. We have examined in past chapters, the stress caused by food and chemical allergy conditions. A combination of both forms of stress will cause rapid deterioration in an already failing system. It is therefore essential, that people with food/chemical intolerances avoid all other forms of stress as much as possible. If they do not, recovery will take far longer and, in some cases, it will just not happen, no matter what other positive steps are taken.

Symptoms of stress

Whether the origin be psychological or physiological, or in other words, external or internal, the symptoms of stress will be the same.

Dr Selye, in *The Stress of Life*, describes, what he has observed to be the more typical signs of stress, once it has risen to dangerous levels. He refers to this situation as 'distress'. Sufferers of allergy illness will recognise many of their own symptoms amongst them:

General irritability, hyperexcitation, or depression. This is associated with unusual agressiveness, or passive indolence, depending upon our constitution. It often manifests itself under, what is called, the 'prima donna' complex.

Pounding of the heart. This is an indication of high blood pressure, often caused by stress.

Dryness of the throat and mouth.

Impulsive behaviour and emotional instability.

The overpowering urge to cry or to run and hide.

Inability to concentrate; daydreaming and general disorientation.

Feelings of unreality, weakness or dizziness.

Predilection to become fatigued and loss of the joy of living.

Floating anxiety, that is to say, we are afraid, although we do not know exactly what we are afraid of.

Emotional tension and alertness, feeling of being 'keyed up'.

Trembling and nervous tics.

Tendency to be easily startled by small sounds.

High pitched nervous laughter.

Stuttering and other speech difficulties which are frequently, stress induced.

Bruxism or grinding of the teeth.

Insomnia, which is usually a consequence of being 'keyed up'.

Hypermobility. This is technically called hyperkinesia, an increased tendency to move about without any reason. An inability to take a physically relaxed attitude, sitting quietly in a chair or lying on a sofa.

Sweating. This becomes evident only under considerable stress.

The frequent need to urinate.

Diarrhoea, indigestion, queasiness in the stomach and, sometimes, even vomiting (These are all signs of disturbed gastrointestinal function which, eventually, may lead to such severe diseases of adaptation as peptic ulcers and ulcerative colitis or irritable colon).

Migraine headaches.

Premenstrual tension or missed menstrual cycles, both of which are frequent indicators of severe stress in women.

Pain in the neck or lower back.

Loss of, or excessive, appetite. This shows itself, soon, in alterations of body weight, namely excessive leanness, or obesity. Some people lose their appetite during stress because of gastrointestinal malfunction, whereas others eat excessively.

Increased smoking.

Increased use of legally prescribed drugs, such as tranquillizers or amphetamines.

Alcohol and drug addiction. Like the phenomenon of overeating, increased and excessive alcohol consumption, or the use of various psychotropic drugs, is a common manifestation of exposure to stresses beyond our natural endurance.

Nightmares.

Neurotic behaviour.

Psychoses.

Accident proneness. Under great stress, we are more likely to have accidents at work, or while driving a car.

Stress threshold

Stress is simply a descriptive term and in itself, not harmful. What is harmful to each individual, is too much stress, or more stress than that particular person can tolerate and still retain good health. This situation is termed by Dr Selye as 'distress' and is the antithesis of 'eustress' or good stress. Distress comes about when the body has been subjected to too much stress, over too long a period. It can no longer recover properly from stress, its biochemical processes have become distorted and it is constantly fatigued. This is a situation of great danger and, if left unattended, will result in chronic illness, followed by disease and death. Dr James Paget, the emminent British physician, has said, 'Fatigue has a larger share in the promotion and transmission of disease than any other single condition you can name'.

Every individual has a different fatigue level or, to put it more appropriately a 'stress threshold'. Dr Selye makes an important statement when he says nobody knows your stress threshold better than you do. It is up to each of us to take careful note of this and live within our personal stress threshold. This can only come about by minimising negative confrontations with daily events and avoiding, whenever possible, allergenic foods and chemicals. In addition, the body can tolerate stress much better if it has an adequate supply of nutrients. It is well known that, in times of stress, the body needs much, much more of these things than at other times. Therefore, increased daily dosages of enzymes, vitamins, minerals and amino acids will greatly help your body's ability to resist stress.

It is particularly important to be aware of your body's daily performance. If you are feeling below par, recognize that fact and do something about it. Daily observation of your stress load can be more important than daily observation of your weight. There are times when we are forced to go through periods of distress. We may not be able to avoid a particular event, but we can avoid other forms of stress during that time by keeping as calm as possible, getting extra sleep and rest, watching what we eat and drink and taking nutrient supplements. Responsible management of ourselves, in this manner, will minimise the degenerative effects that distress has on the body and will enable us to live longer and healthier lives.

Stress and disease

Dr Philpott refers to the stress on the body, from allergic reactions to foods and chemicals, as being the 'central stress building blocks from which many degenerative diseases are constructed'. He says the frequency with which a food is eaten, plus the nutritional quality of the food, determines whether it becomes a stress burden on the metabolic process or not. He reveals that the stress of imbalances in blood sugar levels, insulin production, acid base, and pancreatic enzyme and bicarbonate production, after exposure to allergenic substances, leads to the pancreas being the first organ to develop inhibited function from these stresses. This can result in hypoglycaemia and diabetes.

A further by-product of a malfunctioning pancreas is its tendency to overcompensate for stress-caused high blood sugar, by manufacturing too much insulin. Doctors Meyer Friedman and Ray Rosenman, of San Francisco, comment on this problem in their book, *Type A Behaviour and Your Heart*: 'Of all known conditions that may lead to the disease of coronary arteries, none is recognized as more devastating than any state associated with an excess of insulin in the blood.'

Dr Philpott goes on to say that an overstressed pancreas, should be considered as the foundation of many degenerative diseases. An insufficient supply of pancreatic bicarbonate results in metabolic acidosis in the intestine. As a result, proteolytic enzymes are destroyed and, partly digested, and undigested, proteins (peptides) are absorbed into the blood and evoke kinin-inflammatory reactions in various tissue and organ targets. Thus, a stressed pancreas, leads to a chain reaction of inflammation through the body and, in particular, can cause disturbances and disorientation in the brain. In addition, a stressed pancreas results in amino acid deficiency, which is catastrophic to the nervous system and to many other biochemical functions. A further problem is lowered lipase activity, resulting in a reduced ability to metabolise fats. This, in turn, will cause the body cells to react in a more sensitive fashion to allergenic foods and chemicals.

As a result of these stress-caused biochemical changes, the body is thrown into turmoil and a series of chain reactions results in multiple deficiencies, each feeding off the other. This leads to chronic illness and, finally, major degenerative disease. The effect of prolonged stress, from addictive or ongoing food and chemical allergies, is one of the major causes of degenerative disease.

Additional stress from other sources further aggravates the situation and accelerates a decline in health. Irrespective of the source of stress, the resultant destructive effect on the body's chemistry is the same. We should all make careful assessment of our individual stress threshold and try to live within that limitation. Allergy sufferers, in particular, should be wary of additional stress.

21

CONCLUSION

For a variety of reasons, the human body, during the past few decades, has become increasingly sensitive to our Western lifestyle. Profit–motivated dietary changes, together with chemical pollution of food and environment, have eroded previous standards of health and resilience. Many people are now suffering, unknowingly, from the effects of constant exposure to poorly tolerated foods and chemicals. As a result, the quality of their life has been drastically reduced. Their situation is further aggravated by the fact that modern medical practice has moved away from traditional, healthy methods, of helping the body to overcome illness, to that of poisonous, harmful chemical/drug therapy. Doctors are not taught to understand the relationship of diet and environment to illness, nor to appreciate that organic disease is usually the result of unknowing, and prolonged, auto-intoxication.

In a recent article, in the *New Zealand Medical Journal*, Dr Richard Climie claimed that family doctors will be redundant within ten years, unless drastic changes are made to medical education. According to Dr Climie, medical training is so inadequate for general practice, that the public is now realising it can get better treatment elsewhere. Amongst Dr Climie's comments were: 'People are becoming fed up with pills and outrageous fees. The medical course needed to be drastically changed, with the aim of producing a sensible and competent "generalist".'

With respect to non-medical health practitioners, he said, ' . . . these people have skills that effectively deal with many of the

233

day to day health problems of the population while we still reach for our prescription or referral pad.'

Dr Climie is one of a growing number of doctors who are realizing, that medicine, as it is practised today, is largely ineffective. People are getting fed up with drugs. Often the side effects are worse than the symptoms. Rarely do they cure the underlying cause of the symptom. The move to non-medical health practitioners has been vast during the past decade, as more and more people have been fooled less and less, by the drug-prescription approach. Twenty-four hundred years ago Hippocrates put it in a nutshell, when he said that diet and environment were the key to health. Nothing has changed. That simple truth, if anything, is more valid today than it was then.

There is no doubt that drug therapy saves lives, but at what cost? Often the vicitim has deteriorated, to a point where more and more drugs will be needed to keep him alive. The side effects from these drugs rarely enable him to feel good or lead a normal life. If doctors understood the relationship of diet and environment to illness, they would advise their patients accordingly, and the need for drugs would be dramatically reduced.

There is only one healer, and that is the body itself. Doctors don't heal. Faith healers don't heal. Natural therapists, homeopaths, etc., don't heal. All any health practitioner can do is to try and tip the scales in the sufferer's direction—to take some of the load off the immune system so that the body can take over and heal itself. This is why drugs were originally used, but now they have become something else. Modern drug therapy often seeks to replace immune system function altogether. This does not work. Once the body's natural responses are turned off by drugs, it is often difficult to restart them. There are countless examples of people who have to take drugs permanently, for this reason. There is one sure way to avoid such a situation and that is to examine your diet and environment. Remove the things that are making you sick and you won't need drugs.

The evidence in this book shows beyond any doubt, that many people are suffering from all sorts of distressing symptoms, simply because they are eating or are in contact with substances which have traditionally been considered safe. Furthermore, traditional medical allergy tests have been shown to be virtually useless. Many people now have multiple allergies and, yet, there are very few medical practitioners who can accept this fact — and even fewer who are prepared to do anything about it. Small wonder people are becoming disillusioned and looking elsewhere.

There are signs, however, that attitudes are changing. Several medical school professors have recently spoken of the need for a revision of medical course structure and content, to include more attention to environmental factors. In the meantime, many people will have to be their own physician, until such time as doctors can appreciate that allergies, or intolerances to modern foods and chemicals and the resultant toxic overload to the body, are the cause of a great many, hitherto, unexplained symptoms and illnesses.

BIBLIOGRAPHY

Airola, P., *How to Get Well,* Health Plus, Pheonix Arizona; 1974

Bayly, D., *Reflexology Today,* Thorsons, Wellingborough, Northamptonshire; 1982

Bell, I.R., *Clinical Ecology — A New Medical Approach to Environmental Illness,* Common Knowledge Press, United States; 1982

Bowerman, M. 'Milk and Thought Disorder', *Journal of Orthomolecular Psychiatry,* Vol.9, No.4; 1980

Bright, M., *Living with Your Allergy,* Granada, Richard Clay Ltd, Suffolk; 1982

Bragg, P., 'The Miracle of Fasting', *Health Science;* 1966

Breneman, J., *Basics of Food Allergy,* Charles C. Thomas, Springfield; 1984

Buist,R. *Food Intolerance and How to Cope with It,* Harper & Rowe, Artarmon, New South Wales; 1984

Campbell, M.B., *Allergy of the Nervous System,* Charles C. Thomas, Springfield; 1970

Coca, A.F., *The Pulse Test: Easy Allergy Detection,* Arco Publishing Co, New York; 1972

Colgan, M., *Your Personal Vitamin Profile,* Blond & Briggs Ltd, London; 1983

Collins-Williams, C., *Paediatric Allergy and Clinical Immunology,* Churchill-Livingstone, Edinburgh; 1973

Coeliac Society, *The Coelic Handbook,* The Coeliac Society, London; 1981

Cooper, K.H., *The New Aerobics,* M. Evans & Co, New York; 1977

Crook, W.G., *The Yeast Connection,* Third Edition, 1986. Professional Books and Random House (Vintage Books Division) New York, N.Y.; 1985

Crook, W.G., *Allergy — The Great Masquerader,* Professional Books, Jackson, Tennessee; 1978

Crook, W.G., *Tracking Down Hidden Food Allergy,* Professional Books, Jackson, Tennessee; 1980

Dicky, L.D., (editor), *Clinical Ecology,* Charles C. Thomas, Springfield; 1976

Dumitrescu, I., Edited by Kenyon, J.N., *Electro Graphic Imaging in Medicine and Biology,* Neville Spearman Publications, London; 1983

Eagle, R., *Eating and Allergy,* Future Publications; 1979

Feingold, B.F., *Introduction to Clinical Allergy,* Charles C. Thomas, Springfield; 1973

Feingold, B.F., *Why Your Child is Hyperactive,* Random House, New York; 1974

Frazier, C., *Coping with Food Allergy,* Times Publishing, New York; 1985

Friedman, M., and Rosenman, R., *Type A Behaviour and Your Heart,* Knopf, New York; 1974

Gerard, J., *Food Allergy,* Charles C. Thomas, Springfield; 1980

Goodhart, R.S., and Shils, M.E., *Modern Nutrition in Health and Disease,* Lea & Febiger, Philadelphia; 1980

Hoffer, A., Senility and Chronic Malnutrition, *Journal of Orthomelecular Psychiatry,* Vol.3, No.1, Regina, Saskatchewan; 1974

Hoffer, A., and Walker, M., *Orthomolecular Nutrition,* Keats, New Canaan, Connecticut; 1978

Horne, R., *The New Health Revolution,* Happy Landings Pty. Ltd, Avalon Beach, New South Wales; 1983

Howell, E., *Food Enzymes for Health and Longevity,* Twenty First Century, Fairfield, Iowa; 1981

Hunter, B.T., *Food Additives,* Keats, New Canaan, Connecticut; 1980

Jarrett, R.J., *Nutrition and Disease,* Croom Helm, Beckingham, United Kingdom; 1979

Kenyon, J.N., *Modern Techniques of Acupuncture,* Thorsons Publishers, Wellingborough, Northants; 1983

Kenyon, J.N., 'Measurement in Homoeopathy', *World Medicine,* London; May, 1983

Kenyon, J.N., and Lewith, G.T., 'Ecological Illness — a General Survey', *Medical Paper,* Southampton; 1983

Kenyon, J.N., and Lewith, G.T., 'Immunology in Clinical Ecology', *Medical Paper,* Southampton; 1982

Kenyon, J.N., and Lewith, G.T., 'Rotation Diets', *Medical Paper,* Southampton; 1982

Kenyon, J.N., and Lewith, G.T., 'Chemical and Hydrocarbon Sensitivity', *Medical Paper,* Southampton; 1982

Kenyon, J.N., and Lewith, G.T., 'Electrical Testing as a Means of Diagnosis in Clinical Ecology', *Medical Paper,* Southampton; 1983

Kenyon, J. N., *21st Century Medicine*, Thorsons Publishers, Wellingborough, Northants, 1986

Kenton, L., *Ageless Aging,* Century Publishing, London; 1985

Kingsley, P.J., 'Recognition of Ecological Disease from the History', *Medical Paper,* United Kingdom; 1983

Kingsley, P.J., 'Why and Where the Body has Gone Wrong — The Pancreas, Addiction and Hypoglycaemia', *Medical Paper,* United Kingdom; 1983

Kingsley, P.J., 'The Fast and Reintroduction of Foods', *Medical Paper,* United Kingdom; 1983

Krauze, M.U., and Hunscher, M.A., *Food Nutrition and Diet Therapy,* W.B. Saunders & Co., Philadelphia; 1972

Lessof, M.H., *Clinical Reactions to Food,* John Wiley & Sons, United Kingdom; 1983

Lucas, P., *Clinical Ecology Patients and Candida Albicans,* Germantown, Tennessee; 1982

Mandell, M., *Dr Mandells Five Day Allergy Relief System,* Pocket Books Inc., Division of Simon and Schuster, New York; 1979

Minchin, M., *Food for Thought,* Alma Publications, Melbourne; 1982

Mindell, E., *The Vitamin Bible,* Arlington Books, London; 1982

Montgomery, B., and Evans, L., *You and Stress,* Nelson, Melbourne; 1983

McDonald, A., *Acupuncture: From Ancient Art to Modern Medicine,* Allen & Unwin, London; 1982

Mackarness, R., *Not All in the Mind,* Pan Original, London, 1976

Mackarness, R., *Chemical Victims,* Pan Books, London; 1980

Nutrition Search Inc., *Nutrition Almanac,* McGraw-Hill, New York; 1979

Pauling, L., *Vitamin C and the Common Cold,* W.F. Freeman & Co. San Francisco; 1970

Pfeiffer, C.C., *Zinc and Other Micro-Nutrients,* Keats, New Canaan, Connecticut; 1978

Phillips, D.A., *New Dimension in Health,* Angus & Robertson, Sydney; 1983

Philpott, W., and Kalita, D., *Brain Allergies: The Psychonutrient Connection,* Keats Publishing Inc., New Canaan, Connecticut; 1980

Postma, J.W., *Introduction to the Theory of Physical Education,* A.A. Balkeema, Cape Town; 1980

Pottenger, F.M. Jnr., 'The Effect of Heat-Processed Foods', *American Journal of Orthodontistry and Oral Surgery,* Vol.32, No.8; 1946

Pritikin, N., *The Pritikin Promise,* Bantam Books, New York; 1985

Rapp, D.J., *Allergies and Your Family,* Stirling Publishing, New York; 1980

Randolph, T.G., *Human Ecology and Susceptibility to the Chemical Environment,* Charles C. Thomas, Springfield; 1978

Randolph, T.G., *An Alternative Approach to Allergies,* Harper and Rowe, Scranton; 1980

Rinkel, H.J., Randolph, T.G., and Zeller, M., *Food Allergy,* Charles C. Thomas, Springfield, Illinois; 1951

Reuben, D., *Everything You Always Wanted to Know About Nutrition,* Avon Publishing, New York; 1979

Roe, D.A., *Drug Induced Nutritional Deficiencies,* A.V.I. Publishing, Westport, Connecticut; 1976

Rowe, A.H., and Rowe, A., Jnr., *Food Allergy: Its Manifestations and Control and the Elimination Diets,* Charles C. Thomas, Springfield; 1972

Serizawa, K., *Massage The Oriental Method,* Japan Publications, San Francisco; 1972

Schimmel, H.W., edited by Kenyon, J.N., *Short Manual of the vegatest Method,* VEGA Grieshaber GMBH & Co., Schiltach/ Schwarzwald, West Germany; 1983

Schauss, A., *Diet, Crime and Delinquency,* Parker House, California; 1980

Selye, H., *Stress without Distress: How to Survive in a Stressful Society,* Hodder and Stoughton, London; 1977

Selye, H., *Stress of Life,* McGraw-Hill, New York; 1978. Revised

Smith, L., *Feed Yourself Right,* McGraw-Hill, New York; 1983

Shelton, H.M., *Fasting can Save Your Life,* Natural Hygiene Press, Bridgeport, Connecticut; 1978

Speer, F., *Food Allergy,* P.S.G. Publications, Boston; 1983

Truss, C.O., 'Restoration of Immunologic Competence to Candida Albicans', *The Journal of Orthomolecular Psychiatry,* Vol.9, No.4, Regina, Saskatchewan; 1983

Vayda, W., *Health for Life,* Thomas Nelson Australia, Melbourne; 1981

Vayda, W., 'Crime: Is Nutrition the Missing Link?', *Nature and Health,* Australia; 1983

Vayda, W., 'Do You really need extra Vitamins?', *Australian Well Being,* Sept/Oct; 1984

Walker, N.W., *Colon Health: The Key to a Vibrant Life,* O'Sullivan Woodside & Co., Pheonix, Arizona; 1979

Weiner, M., and Goss, K., *The Complete Book of Homeopathy,* Bantam Books, New York; 1982

Williams, R., *Nutrition Against Disease: Environmental Protection,* Pitman, Marshfield, Massachusetts; 1971

INDEX